DASH DIET COOKBOOK FOR BEGINNERS

2000 Days of Delicious, Nutritious, & Low Sodium Recipes to Help Prevent Hypertension, Lower Your Blood Pressure, and Lose Weight. Includes an 8-Week Meal Plan

Kathleen H. Jensen

CONTENTS

Introduction

Dietary Approaches to Stop Hypertension (DASH) Diet

In this introductory chapter, we will begin our exploration of the DASH Diet. We will learn about its principles, benefits, and the tools necessary to start your culinary adventure.

What is the DASH Diet?

The DASH Diet, which stands for Dietary Approaches to Stop Hypertension, is more than just a diet. It is a lifestyle that focuses on lowering blood pressure and improving cardiovascular health. The DASH Diet is a balanced and nutritious approach to eating that has been developed by nutrition experts and is backed by extensive research. The plan promotes eating whole grains, lean proteins, fruits, and vegetables while advising to limit sodium intake, saturated fats, and sugary treats. As you explore this cookbook, you will find various ways to incorporate the DASH Diet into your daily life, resulting in delicious and satisfying meals.

Benefits of the DASH Diet

The Dietary Approaches to Stop Hypertension (DASH) Diet is a science-backed diet that offers a myriad of health benefits, rather than just being a culinary trend. By adopting the principles of the DASH Diet, you arc not only aiming to reduce your blood pressure, but also starting a journey towards improved overall well-being. Let's explore the various benefits that make the DASH Diet a strong and sustainable option for improving your health.

1. Cardiovascular Health

The DASH Diet has significant effects on cardiovascular health, which is its primary benefit. The DASH Diet is a powerful tool for preventing and managing hypertension by promoting the consumption of nutrient-rich, whole foods and reducing sodium and saturated fat intake. Multiple studies have consistently demonstrated that following the DASH Diet can result in decreased blood pressure levels, thereby reducing the likelihood of developing heart disease and stroke.

2. Weight Management

The DASH Diet is not solely focused on what you should avoid eating; it encourages adopting a balanced and fulfilling approach to nutrition. The DASH Diet emphasizes whole grains, lean proteins, and a variety of fruits and vegetables, which can help with weight management. The fiber and nutrients found in DASH-approved foods can help you feel full and satisfied, and also supports a healthy metabolism.

3. Improved Cholesterol Levels

Manage your cholesterol levels effectively with the DASH Diet. This dietary approach promotes the consumption of heart-healthy fats and foods that are high in soluble fiber, which helps improve the lipid profile. By consuming less saturated fats and foods high in cholesterol, and incorporating more plant-based options into your diet, you can help maintain healthy cholesterol levels and reduce the risk of developing atherosclerosis.

4. Reduced Risk of Chronic Diseases

The DASH Diet has been found to have a positive impact on cardiovascular health and can additionally decrease the risk of chronic diseases. Studies suggest that this dietary approach can have a potential impact on reducing the risk of developing type 2 diabetes, certain cancers, and metabolic syndrome. The DASH Diet includes antioxidant-rich fruits and vegetables that help protect the body from oxidative stress and support overall health.

5. Enhanced Nutrient Intake

One of the notable features of the DASH Diet is its focus on foods that are rich in nutrients. By adopting this eating pattern, you're not only reducing unhealthy choices, but also increasing your intake of vitamins, minerals, and phytonutrients. This not only promotes overall health but also enhances energy levels and cognitive function.

6. Sustainable and Enjoyable

The DASH Diet is sustainable in the long run, unlike many fad diets. The flexibility of this diet allows for a wide variety of foods, making it more enjoyable and sustainable in the long run. The DASH Diet promotes a realistic and enjoyable lifestyle by emphasizing variety, balance, and moderation.

The benefits of the DASH Diet extend beyond blood pressure management. By adopting this holistic approach to eating, you are not only making a dietary change but also investing in a healthier and more vibrant future. The DASH Diet encourages you to improve your well-being by enjoying delicious and nutritious meals.

Chapter 1

Fundamentals of the DASH Diet

The DASH Diet, as earlier stated, is a dietary approach to stop hypertension. It focuses on consuming foods that are low in sodium and high in nutrients like potassium, calcium, and magnesium.

In this chapter, we'll unravel the fundamental principles that define the Dietary Approaches to Stop Hypertension, empowering you to make informed choices that nourish your body and promote overall well-being.

Understanding Dietary Approaches to Stop Hypertension

The DASH Diet is a set of dietary guidelines that have been scientifically proven to reduce blood pressure and promote cardiovascular health. DASH is a balanced diet plan that promotes the consumption of nutrient-dense foods while decreasing the intake of salt, saturated fats, and cholesterol. It was developed by nutrition professionals and is backed by substantial research. Gaining knowledge of DASH's fundamental ideas helps you appreciate its all-encompassing strategy for reaching and preserving a healthy blood pressure level.

Key Principles of the DASH Diet

The DASH Diet is based on several key principles that guide food choices. Among these principles are:

Rich in Fruits and Vegetables: Packed with vital vitamins, minerals, and antioxidants, fruits and vegetables are a great source of nutrition. These elements enhance general immunological function in addition to cardiovascular health.

Emphasis on Whole Grains: The DASH Diet places a strong emphasis on whole grains, including whole wheat, quinoa, and brown rice. These high-fiber grains help to promote digestion, increase satiety, and provide steady energy levels.

Lean Proteins: Choose lean protein sources such as poultry, fish, beans, and tofu. These options provide the necessary amino acids without the saturated fats seen in red meat and processed foods.

Low-Fat Dairy or Non-Dairy Alternatives: Include low-fat dairy products or suitable substitutes in your diet to ensure you are getting enough calcium and vitamin D. These nutrients are very important for keeping your bones healthy.

Healthy Fats: Choose heart-healthy fats such as those found in olive oil, avocados, and nuts. These fats can contribute to overall well-being and add a satisfying element to your meals.

Reduced Sodium Intake: To lower your sodium intake, opt for fresh, unprocessed foods and limit your consumption of packaged and processed items. Managing blood pressure involves controlling sodium intake.

Chapter 2

Getting Started: Essential Kitchen Tools and Ingredients

To start your DASH Diet journey, it's essential to have a well-equipped kitchen that can help you prepare nutritious and tasty meals using wholesome ingredients. Let's discuss the key kitchen tools and ingredients that will enhance your cooking experience and make it more enjoyable.

Essential Kitchen Tools:

1. Quality Chef's Knife: A sharp, high-quality chef's knife is an essential tool for any well-equipped kitchen. The tool makes chopping fruits, vegetables, and lean proteins easier, allowing for precise and efficient meal preparation.

2. Cutting Board: Consider purchasing a cutting board that is durable and easy to clean. Choose one that is wide enough to accommodate several ingredients at once and is made from materials that hinder bacterial growth.

3. Non-Stick Skillet A non-stick skillet is useful for sautéing vegetables and cooking lean proteins with less oil. Select a skillet with a sturdy base to ensure even distribution of heat.

4. Steamer Basket: A steamer basket is a tool used for steaming, which is a common cooking method in the DASH Diet. A steamer basket helps to retain the nutritional value of vegetables while bringing out their natural flavors and colors.

5. Food Processor or Blender: Whether you're making smoothies or whipping up sauces and dips, a food processor or blender can enhance the versatility of your kitchen. This tool is helpful for adding a mix of fruits, vegetables, and nuts to your DASH Diet recipes.

6. Measuring Cups and Spoons: Accurate measurements are necessary for achieving the ideal balance of nutrients in DASH-approved recipes. To ensure precision in your cooking, it is recommended to invest in a set of reliable measuring cups and spoons.

7. Baking Sheets and Pans: Baking sheets and pans are essential for roasting vegetables, baking whole grains, and preparing lean proteins. Select non-stick options for effortless cleaning.

8. Herb and Spice Collection: Complement the flavors of your DASH Diet meals with a thoughtfully selected assortment of herbs and spices. Basil, oregano, cumin, and turmeric are examples of fresh and dried herbs and spices that can enhance the flavor of your dishes without the need for excessive salt.

Essential Ingredients Needed

1. Whole Grains: Stock your pantry with a variety of whole grains like brown rice, quinoa, oats, and whole wheat pasta. Fiber-rich options are a vital component of DASH diet meals.

2. Lean Proteins: Incorporate lean protein sources such as skinless poultry, fish, legumes, tofu, and lean cuts of beef or pork. These proteins offer necessary nutrients without the saturated fats typically present in processed meats.

3. Colorful Vegetables: Include a variety of vegetables in your diet. From leafy greens to colorful bell peppers, these nutrient-rich foods enhance the taste, consistency, and provide an assortment of vitamins to your meals.

4. Fresh Fruits: Have a variety of fresh fruits available for snacking, as well as for desserts and breakfast choices. Berries, apples, citrus fruits, and bananas are great options.

5. Healthy Fats: Introduce heart-healthy fats into your cooking with sources such as olive oil, avocados, and nuts. These fats contribute to satiety and supply vital nutrients for overall health.

6. Low-Fat Dairy or Dairy Alternatives: Choose low-fat dairy products or dairy alternatives such as almond or soy milk. The DASH diet emphasizes bone health and these sources of calcium and vitamin D complement that.

7. Herbs and Spices: Build a collection of herbs and spices to enhance the flavor and complexity of your dishes. Explore different flavors to uncover interesting combinations that can enhance your meals without relying heavily on salt.

By getting these necessary kitchen tools and ingredients, you are setting the groundwork for a successful and enjoyable DASH Diet journey. Having the appropriate equipment and a well-stocked pantry can help you prepare delicious and nutritious meals that support heart-healthy living. Prepare to transform your kitchen into a hub of culinary delights, where you can create delicious and nutritious meals!

Chapter 3: Breakfast

Mediterranean Egg White Omelet

Prep Time: 10 minutes
Cook Time: 10 minutes
Servings: 2

Ingredients:

- 4 large egg whites
- 1/2 cup diced tomatoes
- 1/4 cup chopped spinach
- 1/4 cup chopped bell peppers
- 2 tablespoons diced red onion
- 1/4 cup crumbled feta cheese
- 1/4 teaspoon dried oregano
- 1/4 teaspoon dried basil
- 1/4 teaspoon black pepper
- 1/4 teaspoon olive oil for cooking

Instructions:

1. In a bowl, whisk the egg whites until they are frothy and slightly thickened.

2. Heat the olive oil in a non-stick skillet over medium heat.

3. Add the diced red onion and sauté for 2 minutes or until they become translucent.

4. Stir in the chopped bell peppers and sauté for an additional 2 minutes until they start to soften.

5. Add the diced tomatoes, chopped spinach, dried oregano, and dried basil. Cook for 2-3 minutes until the vegetables are tender.

6. Pour the frothy egg whites over the cooked vegetables in the skillet.

7. Sprinkle the black pepper evenly over the egg whites.

8. Let the omelet cook without stirring for about 5 minutes or until the edges start to set.

9. Sprinkle the crumbled feta cheese evenly over one-half of the omelet.

10. Carefully fold the other half of the omelet over the cheese side to form a half-moon shape.

11. Cook for an additional 2 minutes, allowing the cheese to melt and the omelet to set.

12. Gently slide the omelet onto a plate and serve hot.

Nutritional Information (per serving):

- Carbs: 7 grams

- Fats: 6 grams

- Fiber: 2 grams

- Protein: 18 grams

Quinoa and Spinach Breakfast Bowl

Prep Time: 10 minutes
Cook Time: 20 minutes
Servings: 2

Ingredients:

- 1 cup quinoa

- 2 cups water

- 2 cups fresh spinach, chopped

- 1 cup cherry tomatoes, halved

- 1/2 cup diced cucumber

- 1/4 cup diced red onion

- 1/4 cup crumbled feta cheese

- 2 tablespoons olive oil

- 1 tablespoon lemon juice

- 1/2 teaspoon dried oregano

- Salt and pepper to taste

Instructions:

1. Rinse the quinoa under cold water using a fine mesh strainer.

2. In a medium saucepan, bring two cups of water to a boil.

3. Add the rinsed quinoa to the boiling water. Reduce the heat to low, cover, and simmer for 15-20 minutes, or until the quinoa is tender and the water is absorbed.

4. While the quinoa is cooking, in a large mixing bowl, add the chopped spinach, halved cherry tomatoes, diced cucumber, and diced red onion.

5. In a small bowl, whisk the olive oil, lemon juice, dried oregano, salt, and pepper.

6. When the quinoa is ready, fluff it with a fork and let it cool for a few minutes.

7. Add the cooked quinoa to the bowl of vegetables.

8. Pour the dressing over the quinoa and vegetables and toss to combine.

9. Sprinkle the crumbled feta cheese over the top of the mixture.

10. Serve the Quinoa and Spinach Breakfast Bowl in individual bowls.

Nutritional Information (per serving):

- Carbs: 42 grams

- Fats: 14 grams

- Fiber: 7 grams

- Protein: 12 grams

Avocado and Tomato Breakfast Sandwich

Prep Time: 10 minutes
Cook Time: 5 minutes
Servings: 2

Ingredients:

- 4 slices whole-grain bread

- 1 ripe avocado, mashed

- 1 large tomato, sliced

- 4 large eggs

- 1/4 cup chopped fresh spinach

- 1/4 cup diced red onion

- 1/4 cup low-fat Greek yogurt

- 1/2 teaspoon olive oil

- Salt and pepper to taste

Instructions:

1. Preheat a non-stick skillet over medium heat and add the olive oil.

2. In a bowl, beat the eggs until well combined. Pour the beaten eggs into the skillet.

3. Sprinkle the chopped spinach and diced red onion over the eggs in the skillet.

4. Cook the eggs, spinach, and onion, stirring occasionally, until the eggs are fully cooked and scrambled. Season with salt and pepper to taste.

5. While the eggs are cooking, toast the whole-grain bread slices.

6. Once the eggs are cooked, take them out of the skillet.

7. Spread the mashed avocado onto two slices of the toasted bread.

8. Place the sliced tomato on the other two slices of toasted bread.

9. Divide the scrambled egg mixture evenly between the avocado-topped and tomato-topped slices.

10. Top each sandwich with a dollop of low-fat Greek yogurt.

11. Close the sandwiches by placing the avocado-topped slices on top of the tomato-topped slices.

12. Serve the Avocado and Tomato Breakfast Sandwiches while they are still warm.

Nutritional Information (per serving):

- Carbs: 40 grams

- Fats: 19 grams

- Fiber: 10 grams

- Protein: 18 grams

Sweet Potato and Black Bean Breakfast Tacos

Prep Time: 15 minutes
Cook Time: 20 minutes
Servings: 4

Ingredients:

- 2 cups sweet potatoes, peeled and diced

- 1 can (15 oz) black beans, drained and rinsed

- 8 small whole-grain tortillas
- 4 large eggs
- 1/2 cup diced red bell pepper
- 1/4 cup diced red onion
- 1/4 cup chopped fresh cilantro
- 2 tablespoons olive oil
- 1 teaspoon ground cumin
- 1/2 teaspoon chili powder
- Salt and pepper to taste

Instructions:

1. In a large skillet, heat one tablespoon of olive oil over medium heat.

2. Add the diced sweet potatoes and season with ground cumin, chili powder, salt, and pepper. Sauté until the sweet potatoes are tender, about 10-12 minutes.

3. While the sweet potatoes are cooking, in a separate skillet, heat the remaining olive oil over medium heat.

4. Add the diced red bell pepper and red onion to the skillet. Sauté until they become tender, about 5 minutes.

5. In a small bowl, beat the eggs and pour them into the skillet with the sautéed bell pepper and onion.

6. Cook the eggs, stirring occasionally, until they are fully scrambled and cooked to your desired level of doneness.

7. In a separate pan, heat the black beans until they are warmed through.

8. Warm the whole-grain tortillas in the oven or on a stovetop griddle.

9. To assemble the breakfast tacos, place a portion of the sautéed sweet potatoes on each tortilla.

10. Top with scrambled eggs, black beans, and a sprinkle of fresh cilantro.

11. Fold the tortillas over the filling to create tacos.

12. Serve the Sweet Potato and Black Bean Breakfast Tacos hot.

Nutritional Information (per serving):

- Carbs: 49 grams

- Fats: 12 grams

- Fiber: 11 grams

- Protein: 13 grams

Blueberry Chia Pudding

Prep Time: 5 minutes (plus chilling time)
Cook Time: 0 minutes
Servings: 4

Ingredients:

- 1 cup fresh or frozen blueberries

- 1/4 cup chia seeds

- 2 cups low-fat milk (such as skim or 1% milk)

- 2 tablespoons honey (or to taste)

- 1/2 teaspoon vanilla extract

- 1/4 teaspoon ground cinnamon

- Fresh blueberries and mint leaves for garnish (optional)

Instructions:

1. In a blender, add the fresh or frozen blueberries, low-fat milk, honey, vanilla extract, and ground cinnamon.

2. Blend the ingredients until the mixture is smooth and well combined.

3. In a mixing bowl, pour the blueberry mixture over the chia seeds. Stir to combine.

4. Cover the bowl and refrigerate for at least 4 hours or overnight. This allows the chia seeds to absorb the liquid and thicken.

5. Before serving, give the chia pudding a good stir to make sure the chia seeds are evenly distributed and there are no lumps.

6. Serve the Blueberry Chia Pudding in individual bowls or glasses.

7. If desired, garnish with fresh blueberries and mint leaves for a fresh touch.

Nutritional Information (per serving):

- Carbs: 28 grams
- Fats: 4 grams
- Fiber: 7 grams
- Protein: 6 grams

Greek Yogurt Parfait with Honey and Berries

Prep Time: 10 minutes
Cook Time: 0 minutes
Servings: 2

Ingredients:

- 1 cup low-fat Greek yogurt
- 1 cup mixed berries (e.g., strawberries, blueberries, raspberries)
- 2 tablespoons honey

- 1/4 cup granola

- 1/4 teaspoon vanilla extract

- Fresh mint leaves for garnish (optional)

Instructions:

1. In a bowl, add the low-fat Greek yogurt and vanilla extract. Mix sufficiently to incorporate the vanilla flavor.

2. Wash and prepare the mixed berries as needed. If using strawberries, slice them.

3. In serving glasses or bowls, begin by layering the Greek yogurt mixture. Add a portion of yogurt to the bottom of each glass.

4. Top the yogurt with a layer of mixed berries.

5. Drizzle one tablespoon of honey over the berries in each glass.

6. Add an extra layer of Greek yogurt on top of the honey and berries.

7. Sprinkle granola over the yogurt layer.

8. Drizzle the remaining honey over the granola.

9. If desired, garnish with fresh mint leaves for a pop of color and freshness.

10. Serve the Greek Yogurt Parfait with Honey and Berries immediately.

Nutritional Information (per serving):

- Carbs: 40 grams

- Fats: 3 grams

- Fiber: 4 grams

- Protein: 15 grams

Zucchini and Feta Breakfast Muffins

Prep Time: 15 minutes
Cook Time: 25 minutes
Servings: 6

Ingredients:

- 1 cup grated zucchini (about 1 medium zucchini)
- 1/2 cup crumbled feta cheese
- 1/4 cup diced red bell pepper
- 1/4 cup diced red onion
- 1/4 cup chopped fresh spinach
- 4 large eggs
- 1/4 cup whole-wheat flour
- 1/2 teaspoon baking powder
- 1/4 teaspoon dried oregano
- 1/4 teaspoon dried basil
- Salt and pepper to taste

Instructions:

1. Preheat your oven to 350°F (175°C). Grease a muffin tin or use paper liners.

2. Place the grated zucchini in a clean kitchen towel or paper towels and squeeze to remove excess moisture.

3. In a mixing bowl, add the squeezed zucchini, crumbled feta cheese, diced red bell pepper, diced red onion, and chopped fresh spinach.

4. In a separate bowl, beat the eggs.

5. Stir the beaten eggs into the vegetable mixture.

6. In a small bowl, mix the whole-wheat flour, baking powder, dried oregano, dried basil, salt, and pepper.

7. Gradually add the dry ingredient mixture to the egg and vegetable mixture, stirring until well combined.

8. Divide the mixture evenly among the muffin cups in the prepared tin.

9. Bake in the preheated oven for about 20-25 minutes or until the muffins are set and the tops are lightly golden.

10. Allow the muffins to cool for a few minutes in the tin, then transfer them to a wire rack to cool completely.

11. Serve the Zucchini and Feta Breakfast Muffins warm or at room temperature.

Nutritional Information (per serving):

- Carbs: 8 grams

- Fats: 8 grams

- Fiber: 1 gram

- Protein: 9 grams

Banana Walnut Pancakes

Prep Time: 10 minutes
Cook Time: 15 minutes
Servings: 4

Ingredients:

- 2 ripe bananas, mashed

- 1 1/2 cups whole-wheat flour

- 2 teaspoons baking powder

- 1/2 teaspoon ground cinnamon

- 1/4 teaspoon salt

- 1 1/4 cups low-fat milk

- 2 large eggs

- 1/2 cup chopped walnuts

- 1 tablespoon honey

- 1/2 teaspoon vanilla extract

- Cooking spray or a small amount of vegetable oil for greasing the skillet

Instructions:

1. In a mixing bowl, add the mashed bananas, low-fat milk, eggs, honey, and vanilla extract. Mix sufficiently.

2. In a separate bowl, whisk the whole-wheat flour, baking powder, ground cinnamon, and salt.

3. Gradually add the dry ingredients to the banana mixture, stirring until just combined. Be careful not to overmix; it's okay if there are a few lumps.

4. Gently fold in the chopped walnuts.

5. Preheat a non-stick skillet or griddle over medium heat and lightly grease it with cooking spray or a small amount of vegetable oil.

6. For each pancake, pour approximately 1/4 cup of batter onto the skillet.

7. Cook the pancakes until bubbles form on the surface and the edges start to set, about 2-3 minutes.

8. Flip the pancakes and cook the other side until they are golden brown and cooked through, about 1-2 minutes more.

9. Take out the pancakes from the skillet and keep them warm. Repeat the process with the remaining batter.

10. Serve the Banana Walnut Pancakes with your choice of toppings, such as fresh fruit, a drizzle of honey, or a dollop of Greek yogurt, if desired.

Nutritional Information (per serving):

- Carbs: 45 grams

- Fats: 15 grams

- Fiber: 6 grams

- Protein: 11 grams

Smoked Salmon and Cucumber Toast

Prep Time: 10 minutes
Cook Time: 0 minutes
Servings: 2

Ingredients:

- 4 slices whole-grain bread

- 4 oz smoked salmon

- 1/2 cucumber, thinly sliced

- 2 tablespoons low-fat cream cheese

- 1 tablespoon fresh dill, chopped

- 1/2 lemon, cut into wedges

- Salt and pepper to taste

Instructions:

1. Toast the slices of whole-grain bread to your desired level of crispness.

2. Spread one tablespoon of low-fat cream cheese on each slice of toasted bread.

3. Lay the thinly sliced cucumber on top of the cream cheese on each slice of bread.

4. Divide the smoked salmon into equal portions and drape it over the cucumber slices on each piece of toast.

5. Sprinkle the chopped fresh dill evenly over the smoked salmon.

6. Season with a pinch of salt and a dash of pepper to taste.

7. Serve the Smoked Salmon and Cucumber Toast with lemon wedges on the side for a refreshing squeeze of lemon juice, if desired.

Nutritional Information (per serving):

- Carbs: 35 grams

- Fats: 7 grams

- Fiber: 7 grams

- Protein: 21 grams

Oatmeal with Almond Butter and Apples

Prep Time: 5 minutes
Cook Time: 10 minutes
Servings: 2

Ingredients:

- 1 cup old-fashioned oats

- 2 cups low-fat milk

- 1 apple, peeled, cored, and diced

- 2 tablespoons almond butter

- 1/2 teaspoon ground cinnamon

- 1/4 teaspoon vanilla extract

- 1 tablespoon honey

- 2 tablespoons chopped almonds (optional)

- Fresh apple slices for garnish (optional)

Instructions:

1. In a medium saucepan, add the old-fashioned oats and low-fat milk.

2. Place the saucepan over medium heat and bring the mixture to a boil, stirring occasionally.

3. Reduce the heat to low and add the diced apple to the oatmeal. Simmer for about 5-7 minutes, or until the apples are tender and the oatmeal is creamy, stirring occasionally.

4. Stir in the almond butter, ground cinnamon, and vanilla extract. Mix until the almond butter is fully incorporated, and the oatmeal is well flavored.

5. Take out the oatmeal from the heat and stir in the honey.

6. Serve the Oatmeal with Almond Butter and Apples in bowls. If desired, garnish with chopped almonds and fresh apple slices for extra crunch and flavor.

Nutritional Information (per serving):

- Carbs: 53 grams

- Fats: 15 grams

- Fiber: 7 grams

- Protein: 12 grams

Spinach and Mushroom Frittata

Prep Time: 10 minutes
Cook Time: 20 minutes
Servings: 4

Ingredients:

- 8 large eggs

- 2 cups fresh spinach, chopped

- 1 cup sliced mushrooms

- 1/2 cup diced onion

- 1/2 cup low-fat shredded cheddar cheese

- 2 tablespoons olive oil

- 1/4 teaspoon dried thyme

- Salt and pepper to taste

Instructions:

1. Preheat your oven's broiler.

2. In a large oven-safe skillet, heat the olive oil over medium heat.

3. Add the diced onion and sliced mushrooms to the skillet. Sauté for about 5 minutes or until the mushrooms are tender.

4. Stir in the chopped fresh spinach and cook for an additional 2 minutes until it wilts.

5. In a mixing bowl, beat the eggs and add the dried thyme, salt, and pepper. Mix sufficiently.

6. Pour the beaten egg mixture over the sautéed vegetables in the skillet.

7. Sprinkle the low-fat shredded cheddar cheese evenly over the egg and vegetable mixture.

8. Cook the frittata on the stovetop for about 5 minutes or until the edges start to set.

9. Transfer the skillet to the preheated broiler and cook for an additional 3-5 minutes, until the frittata is set, puffed, and lightly browned on top.

10. Carefully take out the skillet from the oven (use oven mitts as the handle will be hot).

11. Allow the frittata to cool for a few minutes before slicing it into wedges.

12. Serve your Spinach and Mushroom Frittata hot or at room temperature.

Nutritional Information (per serving):

- Carbs: 4 grams

- Fats: 15 grams

- Fiber: 1 gram

- Protein: 13 grams

Breakfast Quinoa with Poached Eggs

Prep Time: 10 minutes
Cook Time: 20 minutes
Servings: 4

Ingredients:

- 1 cup quinoa

- 2 cups low-sodium vegetable broth

- 4 large eggs

- 1 cup diced tomatoes

- 1/2 cup diced red bell pepper

- 1/2 cup chopped fresh spinach

- 1/4 cup diced red onion

- 1/4 cup low-fat feta cheese

- 1 tablespoon olive oil

- 1/2 teaspoon dried oregano

- Salt and pepper to taste

Instructions:

1. Rinse the quinoa under cold water using a fine mesh strainer.

2. In a medium saucepan, bring two cups of low-sodium vegetable broth to a boil.

3. Add the rinsed quinoa to the boiling broth. Reduce the heat to low, cover, and simmer for 15-20 minutes, or until the quinoa is tender and the liquid is absorbed.

4. While the quinoa is cooking, in a separate skillet, heat the olive oil over medium heat.

5. Add the diced red onion and sauté for 2 minutes or until they become translucent.

6. Stir in the diced red bell pepper and sauté for an additional 2 minutes until they start to soften.

7. Add the diced tomatoes and chopped fresh spinach, and cook for 2-3 minutes until the vegetables are tender.

8. Stir in the dried oregano, salt, and pepper.

9. In a separate pot, poach the eggs to your desired level of doneness.

10. To assemble the breakfast bowls, divide the cooked quinoa among four bowls.

11. Top with the sautéed vegetable mixture.

12. Place a poached egg on top of each bowl.

13. Sprinkle low-fat feta cheese evenly over the bowls.

14. Serve your Breakfast Quinoa with Poached Eggs hot and enjoy.

Nutritional Information (per serving):

- Carbs: 35 grams

- Fats: 9 grams

- Fiber: 6 grams

- Protein: 14 grams

Whole Wheat Banana Nut Waffles

Prep Time: 15 minutes
Cook Time: 15 minutes
Servings: 4

Ingredients:

- 1 1/2 cups whole-wheat flour
- 2 teaspoons baking powder
- 1/2 teaspoon ground cinnamon
- 1/4 teaspoon salt
- 2 ripe bananas, mashed
- 1 1/4 cups low-fat milk
- 2 large eggs
- 1/4 cup chopped walnuts
- 1 tablespoon honey
- Cooking spray or a small amount of vegetable oil for greasing the waffle iron

Instructions:

1. Preheat your waffle iron according to the manufacturer's instructions.

2. In a mixing bowl, add the whole-wheat flour, baking powder, ground cinnamon, and salt.

3. In a separate bowl, beat the eggs and add the mashed bananas, low-fat milk, and honey. Mix sufficiently.

4. Pour the wet ingredients into the dry ingredients and stir until just combined. Be careful not to overmix; it's okay if there are a few lumps.

5. Gently fold in the chopped walnuts.

6. Lightly grease the waffle iron with cooking spray or a small amount of vegetable oil.

7. Pour the waffle batter onto the hot waffle iron according to your waffle iron's instructions.

8. Close the waffle iron and cook until the waffles are golden brown and crisp, about 5-7 minutes.

9. Carefully take out the waffles from the iron and keep them warm.

10. Repeat the process with the remaining batter.

11. Serve the Whole Wheat Banana Nut Waffles hot with your choice of toppings, such as fresh fruit or a drizzle of honey.

Nutritional Information (per serving):

- Carbs: 49 grams

- Fats: 12 grams

- Fiber: 6 grams

- Protein: 11 grams

Cherry Almond Breakfast Bars

Prep Time: 15 minutes
Cook Time: 30 minutes
Servings: 12

Ingredients:

- 2 cups old-fashioned oats

- 1 cup whole-wheat flour

- 1/2 cup unsalted almonds, chopped

- 1/2 cup dried cherries, chopped

- 1/2 cup low-fat milk

- 1/4 cup honey

- 1/4 cup unsweetened applesauce

- 1/4 cup almond butter

- 1 large egg

- 1 teaspoon vanilla extract

- 1/2 teaspoon ground cinnamon

- 1/4 teaspoon salt

Instructions:

1. Preheat your oven to 350°F (175°C). Grease or line a 9x9-inch (23x23 cm) baking pan.

2. In a large mixing bowl, add the old-fashioned oats, whole-wheat flour, chopped unsalted almonds, and chopped dried cherries.

3. In a separate microwave-safe bowl, heat the almond butter until it's easier to stir, about 20-30 seconds.

4. Add the low-fat milk, honey, unsweetened applesauce, almond butter, egg, vanilla extract, ground cinnamon, and salt to the dry ingredients in the large bowl. Mix until everything is well combined.

5. Press the mixture into the prepared baking pan, spreading it evenly.

6. Bake in the preheated oven for approximately 25-30 minutes or until the bars are set and the edges are lightly golden.

7. Take out the bars from the oven and allow them to cool in the pan.

8. Once cooled, cut the Cherry Almond Breakfast Bars into 12 servings.

Nutritional Information (per serving):

- Carbs: 32 grams

- Fats: 9 grams

- Fiber: 4 grams

- Protein: 7 grams

Coconut Mango Smoothie Bowl

Prep Time: 10 minutes
Cook Time: 0 minutes
Servings: 2

Ingredients:

- 2 cups frozen mango chunks

- 1 cup low-fat Greek yogurt

- 1/2 cup unsweetened coconut milk

- 1/4 cup unsweetened shredded coconut

- 1 tablespoon honey

- 1/4 teaspoon vanilla extract

- Sliced fresh mango, kiwi, and berries for topping

- Chopped nuts (e.g., almonds or walnuts) for topping (optional)

Instructions:

1. In a blender, add the frozen mango chunks, low-fat Greek yogurt, unsweetened coconut milk, unsweetened shredded coconut, honey, and vanilla extract.

2. Blend the ingredients until the mixture is smooth and has a thick, smoothie-like consistency.

3. If the mixture is too thick, you can add a little more coconut milk to achieve the desired consistency.

4. Pour the coconut mango smoothie into two serving bowls.

5. Top each bowl with sliced fresh mango, kiwi, berries, and chopped nuts, if desired.

6. Serve your Coconut Mango Smoothie Bowl immediately.
Nutritional Information (per serving):

- Carbs: 39 grams

- Fats: 7 grams

- Fiber: 4 grams

- Protein: 11 grams

Spinach and Mushroom Breakfast Quesadilla

Prep Time: 15 minutes
Cook Time: 15 minutes
Servings: 2

Ingredients:

- 4 large whole-wheat tortillas

- 2 cups fresh spinach

- 1 cup sliced mushrooms

- 1/2 cup diced red bell pepper

- 1/4 cup diced red onion

- 1/2 cup low-fat shredded cheddar cheese

- 4 large eggs

- 2 tablespoons low-fat milk

- 1/2 teaspoon dried oregano

- 1/2 teaspoon dried basil

- 1/4 teaspoon garlic powder

- Salt and pepper to taste

- Cooking spray or a small amount of vegetable oil for greasing the skillet

Instructions:

1. In a skillet, heat a small amount of vegetable oil or use cooking spray and sauté the diced red onion until it becomes translucent.

2. Add the sliced mushrooms and diced red bell pepper to the skillet. Sauté for about 5 minutes or until the vegetables are tender.

3. Stir in the fresh spinach and cook for an additional 2-3 minutes until it wilts. Set the cooked vegetables aside.

4. In a bowl, beat the eggs and add the low-fat milk, dried oregano, dried basil, garlic powder, salt, and pepper. Mix sufficiently.

5. Heat a non-stick skillet over medium heat and add a tortilla to the skillet.

6. Sprinkle half of the low-fat shredded cheddar cheese evenly over the tortilla.

7. Pour half of the egg mixture over the cheese.

8. Spread half of the sautéed vegetable mixture over the eggs.

9. Place an extra tortilla on top and press down gently.

10. Cook until the bottom tortilla is golden brown, then carefully flip the quesadilla and cook the other side until it's golden brown and the cheese is melted.

11. Repeat the process for the second quesadilla.

12. Slice each quesadilla into quarters, creating four wedges per quesadilla.

13. Serve your Spinach and Mushroom Breakfast Quesadilla hot.

Nutritional Information (per serving):

- Carbs: 43 grams

- Fats: 15 grams

- Fiber: 7 grams

- Protein: 24 grams

Cinnamon Raisin Oatmeal with Sliced Apples

Prep Time: 5 minutes
Cook Time: 10 minutes
Servings: 2

Ingredients:

- 1 cup old-fashioned oats

- 2 cups low-fat milk

- 1 apple, peeled, cored, and sliced

- 1/4 cup raisins

- 1/2 teaspoon ground cinnamon

- 1/4 teaspoon vanilla extract

- 1 tablespoon honey

- A pinch of salt

- Chopped nuts (e.g., almonds or walnuts) for garnish (optional)

Instructions:

1. In a saucepan, add the old-fashioned oats, low-fat milk, sliced apple, raisins, ground cinnamon, vanilla extract, honey, and a pinch of salt.

2. Place the saucepan over medium heat and bring the mixture to a boil.

3. Reduce the heat to low and simmer for about 5-7 minutes, or until the oats are tender and the mixture thickens, stirring occasionally.

4. If the oatmeal becomes too thick, you can add a little more milk to reach your desired consistency.

5. Take out the oatmeal from the heat.

6. Serve your Cinnamon Raisin Oatmeal with Sliced Apples in bowls.

7. If desired, garnish with chopped nuts for added texture and flavor.

Nutritional Information (per serving):

- Carbs: 60 grams

- Fats: 6 grams

- Fiber: 7 grams

- Protein: 11 grams

Smoked Salmon and Asparagus Frittata

Prep Time: 10 minutes
Cook Time: 20 minutes
Servings: 4

Ingredients:

- 8 large eggs

- 8 asparagus spears, trimmed and sliced into 1-inch pieces

- 4 oz smoked salmon, cut into small pieces

- 1/2 cup low-fat cream cheese

- 1/4 cup chopped fresh dill

- 1/4 cup diced red onion

- 1/4 teaspoon black pepper

- 1/4 teaspoon salt

- Cooking spray or a small amount of vegetable oil for greasing the skillet

Instructions:

1. Preheat your oven's broiler.

2. In a mixing bowl, beat the eggs.

3. Stir in the chopped fresh dill, diced red onion, black pepper, and salt.

4. Heat an oven-safe skillet over medium heat and lightly grease it with cooking spray or a small amount of vegetable oil.

5. Add the sliced asparagus to the skillet and sauté for about 3 minutes, or until they are slightly tender.

6. Spread the asparagus evenly in the skillet and distribute the smoked salmon pieces on top.

7. Pour the beaten egg mixture over the asparagus and salmon.

8. Dot the low-fat cream cheese over the top of the frittata.

9. Cook on the stovetop for about 5 minutes or until the edges start to set.

10. Transfer the skillet to the preheated broiler and cook for an additional 3-5 minutes until the frittata is set and lightly browned on top.

11. Carefully take out the skillet from the oven (use oven mitts as the handle will be hot).

12. Allow the frittata to cool for a few minutes before slicing it into wedges.

13. Serve your Smoked Salmon and Asparagus Frittata hot and enjoy.

Nutritional Information (per serving):

- Carbs: 2 grams

- Fats: 11 grams

- Fiber: 1 gram

- Protein: 17 grams

Banana and Walnut Breakfast Quinoa

Prep Time: 10 minutes
Cook Time: 15 minutes
Servings: 2

Ingredients:

- 1 cup quinoa
- 2 cups low-fat milk
- 2 ripe bananas, sliced
- 1/4 cup chopped walnuts
- 2 tablespoons honey
- 1/2 teaspoon ground cinnamon
- 1/4 teaspoon vanilla extract
- A pinch of salt

Instructions:

1. Rinse the quinoa under cold water using a fine mesh strainer.

2. In a medium saucepan, bring two cups of low-fat milk to a boil.

3. Add the rinsed quinoa to the boiling milk. Reduce the heat to low, cover, and simmer for 12-15 minutes, or until the quinoa is tender and the liquid is absorbed.

4. While the quinoa is cooking, in a separate bowl, add the sliced bananas, chopped walnuts, honey, ground cinnamon, vanilla extract, and a pinch of salt.

5. When the quinoa is cooked, fluff it with a fork and then fold in the banana and walnut mixture. Allow it to sit for a minute to warm the bananas and add the flavors.

6. Serve your Banana and Walnut Breakfast Quinoa hot.

Nutritional Information (per serving):

- Carbs: 60 grams

- Fats: 11 grams

- Fiber: 6 grams

- Protein: 12 grams

Greek Yogurt with Berries and Chia Seeds

Prep Time: 5 minutes
Cook Time: 0 minutes
Servings: 2

Ingredients:

- 2 cups low-fat Greek yogurt

- 1 cup mixed berries (e.g., blueberries, strawberries, raspberries)

- 2 tablespoons chia seeds

- 2 tablespoons honey

- 1/2 teaspoon vanilla extract

Instructions:

1. In a mixing bowl, add the low-fat Greek yogurt, chia seeds, honey, and vanilla extract.

2. Stir the mixture thoroughly to evenly distribute the chia seeds.

3. In serving bowls or glasses, layer the chia seed yogurt mixture and mixed berries.

4. Repeat the layering process until the bowls or glasses are filled.

5. Top each serving with an extra drizzle of honey, if desired.

6. Serve your Greek Yogurt with Berries and Chia Seeds immediately.

Nutritional Information (per serving):

- Carbs: 36 grams

- Fats: 6 grams

- Fiber: 8 grams

- Protein: 18 grams

Sweet Potato and Kale Breakfast Hash

Prep Time: 10 minutes
Cook Time: 20 minutes
Servings: 2

Ingredients:

- 2 cups sweet potatoes, peeled and diced

- 2 cups kale, chopped

- 1/2 cup red bell pepper, diced

- 1/2 cup red onion, diced

- 2 large eggs

- 1 tablespoon olive oil

- 1/2 teaspoon paprika

- 1/2 teaspoon garlic powder

- 1/4 teaspoon black pepper

- A pinch of salt

- Cooking spray or a small amount of vegetable oil for greasing the skillet

Instructions:

1. In a skillet, heat the olive oil over medium heat.

2. Add the diced sweet potatoes and cook for about 10-12 minutes, or until they are tender and lightly browned, stirring occasionally. Cover the skillet to help them cook faster.

3. Stir in the diced red bell pepper and cook for an additional 2 minutes.

4. Add the diced red onion and continue to cook for an extra 2 minutes, or until the onion is soft and translucent.

5. Sprinkle the paprika, garlic powder, black pepper, and a pinch of salt over the sweet potato mixture. Stir to add and let it cook for an extra 2 minutes.

6. Add the chopped kale to the skillet and cook for 3-4 minutes, or until it's wilted and tender.

7. Create two small wells in the hash, and crack an egg into each well.

8. Cover the skillet and cook for about 4-5 minutes, or until the egg whites are set but the yolks are still slightly runny. Cook longer if you prefer your eggs more well-done.

9. Carefully take out the skillet from the heat.

10. Serve your Sweet Potato and Kale Breakfast Hash hot, dividing it into two portions.

Nutritional Information (per serving):

- Carbs: 39 grams

- Fats: 14 grams

- Fiber: 6 grams

- Protein: 11 grams

Mango and Coconut Chia Pudding

Prep Time: 10 minutes (plus chilling time)
Cook Time: 0 minutes
Servings: 2

Ingredients:

- 1/2 cup chia seeds

- 1 1/2 cups low-fat coconut milk

- 1 ripe mango, diced

- 1 tablespoon honey

- 1/2 teaspoon vanilla extract

- Unsweetened shredded coconut for garnish (optional)

Instructions:

1. In a mixing bowl, add the chia seeds and low-fat coconut milk.

2. Add the honey and vanilla extract to the mixture. Stir sufficiently to combine.

3. Cover the bowl and refrigerate for at least 2 hours or overnight. This allows the chia seeds to absorb the liquid and create a pudding-like consistency.

4. Before serving, dice the ripe mango.

5. To assemble the pudding, divide the chia seed mixture into two serving glasses or bowls.

6. Top the chia pudding with the diced mango.

7. If desired, garnish with unsweetened shredded coconut for added flavor and texture.

8. Serve your Mango and Coconut Chia Pudding cold, and enjoy.

Nutritional Information (per serving):

- Carbs: 41 grams

- Fats: 17 grams

- Fiber: 13 grams

- Protein: 6 grams

Whole Wheat Blueberry Muffins

Prep Time: 15 minutes
Cook Time: 20 minutes
Servings: 12

Ingredients:

- 2 cups whole wheat flour
- 1/2 cup rolled oats
- 1/2 cup honey or maple syrup
- 1/4 cup unsalted butter, melted
- 1 cup low-fat milk
- 2 eggs
- 1 1/2 cups fresh blueberries
- 1 teaspoon baking powder
- 1/2 teaspoon baking soda
- 1/2 teaspoon vanilla extract
- 1/4 teaspoon salt

Instructions:

1. Preheat your oven to 350°F (175°C) and line a muffin tin with paper liners or lightly grease the cups.

2. In a large mixing bowl, add the whole wheat flour, rolled oats, baking powder, baking soda, and salt.

3. In an extra bowl, whisk the melted unsalted butter, honey or maple syrup, low-fat milk, eggs, and vanilla extract.

4. Pour the wet ingredients into the dry ingredients and stir until just combined. Be careful not to overmix; a few lumps are fine.

5. Gently fold in the fresh blueberries.

6. Divide the muffin batter evenly among the prepared muffin cups.

7. Bake in the preheated oven for about 18-20 minutes, or until a toothpick inserted into the center of a muffin comes out clean.

8. Allow the muffins to cool in the tin for a few minutes, then transfer them to a wire rack to cool completely.

9. Serve your Whole Wheat Blueberry Muffins as a delicious DASH diet-friendly breakfast or snack.

Nutritional Information (per muffin):

- Carbs: 32 grams

- Fats: 5 grams

- Fiber: 3 grams

- Protein: 4 grams

Chapter 4: Appetizers & Snacks

Cucumber and Tomato Salsa

Prep Time: 15 minutes
Cook Time: 0 minutes
Number of Servings: 6

Ingredients:

- 2 cups cucumbers, diced
- 2 cups tomatoes, diced
- 1/2 cup red onion, finely chopped
- 1/4 cup fresh cilantro, chopped
- 1 jalapeño pepper, seeds Take outd and finely diced
- 2 cloves garlic, minced
- 2 tablespoons fresh lime juice
- 1/2 teaspoon ground cumin
- 1/2 teaspoon salt
- 1/4 teaspoon black pepper

Instructions:

1. In a large mixing bowl, add the diced cucumbers, diced tomatoes, finely chopped red onion, chopped cilantro, and finely diced jalapeño pepper.

2. In a small bowl, whisk the minced garlic, fresh lime juice, ground cumin, salt, and black pepper.

3. Pour the lime juice mixture over the diced vegetables in the large mixing bowl.

4. Gently toss all the ingredients together until well combined.

5. Refrigerate the salsa for at least 30 minutes before serving to allow the flavors to meld.

6. Serve the DASH-friendly Cucumber and Tomato Salsa as a refreshing side dish or with whole-grain tortilla chips.

Nutritional Information (per serving):

- Carbs: 8g

- Fats: 0g

- Fiber: 2g

- Protein: 1g

Roasted Red Pepper Hummus

Prep Time: 15 minutes
Cook Time: 0 minutes
Number of Servings: 8

Ingredients:

- 1 can (15 ounces) chickpeas, drained and rinsed

- 2/3 cup roasted red peppers, drained and chopped

- 1/4 cup tahini

- 2 tablespoons fresh lemon juice

- 2 cloves garlic, minced

- 1/2 teaspoon ground cumin

- 1/2 teaspoon salt

- 1/4 teaspoon black pepper

- 1 tablespoon extra-virgin olive oil

- 1 tablespoon fresh parsley, chopped (for garnish)

Instructions:

1. In a food processor, add the drained and rinsed chickpeas, chopped roasted red peppers, tahini, fresh lemon juice, minced garlic, ground cumin, salt, and black pepper.

2. Process the mixture until it becomes smooth and creamy, scraping down the sides of the bowl as needed.

3. Transfer the roasted red pepper hummus to a serving bowl.

4. Drizzle the extra-virgin olive oil over the top, and garnish with the chopped fresh parsley.

5. Serve the DASH-friendly Roasted Red Pepper Hummus with whole-grain pita bread, vegetable sticks, or whole-grain crackers.

Nutritional Information (per serving):

- Carbs: 14g

- Fats: 5g

- Fiber: 3g

- Protein: 4g

Spiced Edamame

Prep Time: 10 minutes
Cook Time: 5 minutes
Number of Servings: 4

Ingredients:

- 2 cups edamame (shelled)

- 1 tablespoon olive oil

- 1 teaspoon ground cumin

- 1/2 teaspoon ground coriander

- 1/4 teaspoon ground turmeric

- 1/4 teaspoon paprika

- 1/4 teaspoon salt

- 1/8 teaspoon black pepper

- 1 tablespoon fresh cilantro, chopped (for garnish)

Instructions:

1. In a large pot, bring water to a boil. Add the shelled edamame and cook for 3-5 minutes or until they are tender. Drain the edamame and set them aside.

2. In a large skillet, heat the olive oil over medium heat. Add the ground cumin, ground coriander, ground turmeric, paprika, salt, and black pepper. Stir the spices in the oil for about 1 minute to release their flavors.

3. Add the cooked edamame to the skillet and toss them with the spiced oil mixture. Sauté for an additional 2 minutes to coat the edamame evenly and heat them through.

4. Transfer the spiced edamame to a serving dish and garnish with the chopped fresh cilantro.

5. Serve this DASH-friendly Spiced Edamame as a healthy and flavorful snack or side dish.

Nutritional Information (per serving):

- Carbs: 10g

- Fats: 4g

- Fiber: 4g

- Protein: 7g

Guacamole-Stuffed Mini Peppers

Prep Time: 20 minutes
Cook Time: 0 minutes
Number of Servings: 6

Ingredients:

- 12 mini sweet peppers

- 2 ripe avocados, peeled, pitted, and mashed

- 1/4 cup red onion, finely diced

- 1/4 cup tomato, diced

- 2 tablespoons fresh cilantro, chopped

- 1 clove garlic, minced

- 1/2 lime, juiced

- 1/4 teaspoon salt

- 1/8 teaspoon black pepper

Instructions:

1. Cut the tops off the mini sweet peppers and take out the seeds and membranes.

2. In a mixing bowl, add the mashed avocados, finely diced red onion, diced tomato, chopped fresh cilantro, minced garlic, fresh lime juice, salt, and black pepper. Mix sufficiently to make the guacamole.

3. Using a small spoon, stuff each mini sweet pepper with the prepared guacamole.

4. Arrange the stuffed peppers on a serving platter.

5. Serve these DASH-friendly Guacamole-Stuffed Mini Peppers as a delightful appetizer or snack.

Nutritional Information (per serving):

- Carbs: 10g

- Fats: 7g

- Fiber: 4g

- Protein: 2g

Baked Sweet Potato Fries

Prep Time: 15 minutes
Cook Time: 25 minutes
Number of Servings: 4

Ingredients:

- 2 large sweet potatoes, peeled and cut into 1/4-inch wide strips

- 2 tablespoons olive oil

- 1/2 teaspoon paprika

- 1/2 teaspoon garlic powder

- 1/2 teaspoon onion powder

- 1/4 teaspoon salt

- 1/4 teaspoon black pepper

Instructions:

1. Preheat your oven to 425°F (220°C) and line a baking sheet with parchment paper.

2. In a large bowl, add the sweet potato strips, olive oil, paprika, garlic powder, onion powder, salt, and black pepper. Toss to coat the sweet potato strips evenly with the seasonings and oil.

3. Spread the seasoned sweet potato strips out in a single layer on the prepared baking sheet.

4. Bake in the preheated oven for 20-25 minutes, or until the sweet potato fries are crispy and golden brown, turning them once halfway through the cooking time.

5. Take out the baked sweet potato fries from the oven and let them cool slightly before serving.

6. Serve these DASH-friendly Baked Sweet Potato Fries as a nutritious and tasty side dish or snack.

Nutritional Information (per serving):

- Carbs: 24g

- Fats: 7g

- Fiber: 4g

- Protein: 2g

Tuna Salad Lettuce Wraps

Prep Time: 15 minutes
Cook Time: 0 minutes
Number of Servings: 4

Ingredients:

- 2 cans (5 ounces each) of tuna, drained

- 1/2 cup celery, finely diced

- 1/4 cup red onion, finely diced

- 1/4 cup dill pickles, finely diced

- 1/4 cup mayonnaise

- 1 tablespoon Dijon mustard

- 1/2 teaspoon dried dill

- 1/4 teaspoon black pepper

- 8 large lettuce leaves (such as iceberg or Romaine)

Instructions:

1. In a mixing bowl, add the drained tuna, finely diced celery, finely diced red onion, finely diced dill pickles, mayonnaise, Dijon

mustard, dried dill, and black pepper. Mix the ingredients until well combined to make the tuna salad.

2. Take a large lettuce leaf, and place a scoop of the tuna salad in the center.

3. Fold the sides of the lettuce leaf over the tuna salad and then roll it up to create a lettuce wrap.

4. Repeat this process with the remaining lettuce leaves and tuna salad.

5. Serve these DASH-friendly Tuna Salad Lettuce Wraps as a light and satisfying meal or snack.

Nutritional Information (per serving):

- Carbs: 4g

- Fats: 13g

- Fiber: 1g

- Protein: 17g

Caprese Skewers with Balsamic Glaze

Prep Time: 15 minutes
Cook Time: 5 minutes
Number of Servings: 4

Ingredients:

- 16 cherry tomatoes

- 16 fresh mozzarella balls (mini)

- 16 fresh basil leaves

- 1/4 cup balsamic vinegar

- 1 teaspoon honey

- 1/4 teaspoon salt

- 1/4 teaspoon black pepper

Instructions:

1. In a small saucepan, add the balsamic vinegar and honey. Heat over low heat, stirring occasionally, until the mixture has reduced by half and has a syrupy consistency. This should take about 5 minutes. Take out from heat and let it cool.

2. Assemble the Caprese skewers by threading a cherry tomato, a fresh mozzarella ball, and a fresh basil leaf onto each skewer. Repeat until you have made 16 skewers.

3. Place the assembled skewers on a serving platter.

4. Drizzle the balsamic glaze over the Caprese skewers.

5. Sprinkle the skewers with salt and black pepper.

6. Serve these DASH-friendly Caprese Skewers with Balsamic Glaze as a delightful appetizer or light snack.

Nutritional Information (per serving):

- Carbs: 6g

- Fats: 10g

- Fiber: 0.5g

- Protein: 5g

Chickpea and Spinach Dip
Prep Time: 15 minutes
Cook Time: 5 minutes
Number of Servings: 6

Ingredients:

- 1 can (15 ounces) chickpeas, drained and rinsed

- 2 cups fresh spinach, chopped

- 1/4 cup plain Greek yogurt

- 1/4 cup feta cheese, crumbled

- 1/4 cup olive oil

- 2 cloves garlic, minced

- 1 tablespoon lemon juice

- 1/2 teaspoon ground cumin

- 1/4 teaspoon salt

- 1/4 teaspoon black pepper

Instructions:

1. In a small skillet, heat one tablespoon of olive oil over medium heat. Add the minced garlic and cook for about 1 minute until fragrant. Take out from heat and let it cool.

2. In a food processor, add the chickpeas, chopped fresh spinach, cooled garlic and oil mixture, Greek yogurt, crumbled feta cheese, lemon juice, ground cumin, salt, and black pepper.

3. Process the mixture until it is smooth and creamy, scraping down the sides of the bowl as needed.

4. Transfer the Chickpea and Spinach Dip to a serving bowl.

5. Serve this DASH-friendly Chickpea and Spinach Dip with fresh vegetable sticks or whole-grain crackers.

Nutritional Information (per serving):

- Carbs: 11g

- Fats: 7g

- Fiber: 3g

- Protein: 6g

Greek Salad Bites

Prep Time: 20 minutes
Cook Time: 0 minutes
Number of Servings: 4

Ingredients:

- 1 cucumber, diced into 1/4-inch pieces

- 1 cup cherry tomatoes, quartered

- 1/2 cup red onion, finely diced

- 1/2 cup feta cheese, crumbled

- 1/4 cup Kalamata olives, pitted and sliced

- 2 tablespoons extra-virgin olive oil

- 1 tablespoon fresh lemon juice

- 1 teaspoon dried oregano

- Salt and black pepper to taste

- 16 cucumber or endive leaves (as serving cups)

Instructions:

1. In a mixing bowl, add the diced cucumber, quartered cherry tomatoes, finely diced red onion, crumbled feta cheese, and sliced Kalamata olives.

2. In a separate small bowl, whisk the extra-virgin olive oil, fresh lemon juice, dried oregano, salt, and black pepper to create the dressing.

3. Pour the dressing over the salad mixture and toss to coat the ingredients evenly.

4. Spoon the Greek salad into cucumber or endive leaves, using them as serving cups.

5. Serve these DASH-friendly Greek Salad Bites as a refreshing and healthy appetizer or snack.

Nutritional Information (per serving):

- Carbs: 10g

- Fats: 13g

- Fiber: 3g

- Protein: 4g

Quinoa-Stuffed Mushrooms

Prep Time: 20 minutes
Cook Time: 25 minutes
Number of Servings: 4

Ingredients:

- 8 large mushrooms

- 1 cup quinoa

- 2 cups vegetable broth

- 1/2 cup red bell pepper, finely diced

- 1/4 cup red onion, finely diced

- 1/4 cup fresh parsley, chopped

- 2 cloves garlic, minced

- 1/4 teaspoon dried thyme

- 1/4 teaspoon dried oregano

- 1/4 teaspoon salt

- 1/4 teaspoon black pepper

- 1/4 cup grated Parmesan cheese (optional)

Instructions:

1. Preheat your oven to 375°F (190°C) and line a baking sheet with parchment paper.

2. Clean the mushrooms and take out the stems. Set the caps aside.

3. In a fine-mesh strainer, rinse the quinoa under cold water.

4. In a medium saucepan, bring the vegetable broth to a boil. Add the rinsed quinoa, reduce the heat to a simmer, cover, and cook for about 15 minutes, or until the quinoa is cooked and the liquid is absorbed. Take out from heat.

5. In a large mixing bowl, add the cooked quinoa, finely diced red bell pepper, finely diced red onion, chopped fresh parsley, minced garlic, dried thyme, dried oregano, salt, and black pepper. Mix sufficiently.

6. Stuff each mushroom cap with the quinoa mixture, pressing it in firmly. If desired, sprinkle the stuffed mushrooms with grated Parmesan cheese.

7. Place the stuffed mushrooms on the prepared baking sheet.

8. Bake in the preheated oven for about 20-25 minutes, or until the mushrooms are tender and the stuffing is heated through.

9. Serve these DASH-friendly Quinoa-Stuffed Mushrooms as a satisfying and nutritious appetizer or side dish.

Nutritional Information (per serving):

- Carbs: 31g

- Fats: 5g

- Fiber: 4g

- Protein: 9g

Crispy Kale Chips

Prep Time: 10 minutes
Cook Time: 15 minutes
Number of Servings: 4

Ingredients:

- 1 bunch of fresh kale, stems Take outd and leaves torn into bite-sized pieces
- 2 tablespoons olive oil
- 1/4 teaspoon salt
- 1/4 teaspoon black pepper

Instructions:

1. Preheat your oven to 350°F (175°C) and line a baking sheet with parchment paper.

2. In a large mixing bowl, toss the torn kale leaves with olive oil, ensuring each leaf is lightly coated.

3. Spread the kale leaves in a single layer on the prepared baking sheet.

4. Sprinkle the salt and black pepper evenly over the kale leaves.

5. Bake in the preheated oven for about 12-15 minutes, or until the kale leaves are crisp but not burnt. Keep a close eye on them, as cooking time may vary depending on your oven.

6. Take out the crispy kale chips from the oven and let them cool before serving.

7. Serve these DASH-friendly Crispy Kale Chips as a healthy and guilt-free snack.

Nutritional Information (per serving):

- Carbs: 5g
- Fats: 7g

- Fiber: 1g

- Protein: 2g

Watermelon and Feta Skewers

Prep Time: 15 minutes
Cook Time: 0 minutes
Number of Servings: 4

Ingredients:

- 2 cups watermelon, diced into 1-inch cubes

- 1 cup feta cheese, diced into 1-inch cubes

- 16 fresh basil leaves

- 2 tablespoons balsamic vinegar

- 1 tablespoon extra-virgin olive oil

- 1/4 teaspoon black pepper

- 8 wooden skewers

Instructions:

1. In a small bowl, whisk the balsamic vinegar, extra-virgin olive oil, and black pepper to create a dressing.

2. Assemble the skewers by threading a watermelon cube, a feta cheese cube, and a fresh basil leaf onto each skewer. Repeat until you have made 8 skewers.

3. Place the assembled skewers on a serving platter.

4. Drizzle the balsamic dressing over the Watermelon and Feta Skewers.

5. Serve these DASH-friendly Watermelon and Feta Skewers as a refreshing and delightful appetizer or snack.

Nutritional Information (per serving):

- Carbs: 13g

- Fats: 9g

- Fiber: 1g

- Protein: 7g

Spicy Oven-Baked Sweet Potato Wedges

Prep Time: 15 minutes
Cook Time: 30 minutes
Number of Servings: 4

Ingredients:

- 2 large sweet potatoes, washed and cut into wedges

- 2 tablespoons olive oil

- 1 teaspoon paprika

- 1/2 teaspoon chili powder

- 1/2 teaspoon garlic powder

- 1/2 teaspoon onion powder

- 1/2 teaspoon salt

- 1/4 teaspoon black pepper

- 1/4 teaspoon cayenne pepper (adjust to taste)

- Cooking spray (olive oil or canola oil)

Instructions:

1. Preheat your oven to 425°F (220°C) and line a baking sheet with parchment paper. Lightly coat the parchment paper with cooking spray.

2. In a large mixing bowl, toss the sweet potato wedges with olive oil, ensuring they are evenly coated.

3. In a separate bowl, add paprika, chili powder, garlic powder, onion powder, salt, black pepper, and cayenne pepper. Mix to create a spice blend.

4. Sprinkle the spice blend over the sweet potato wedges and toss to coat them with the spices.

5. Arrange the seasoned sweet potato wedges in a single layer on the prepared baking sheet.

6. Bake in the preheated oven for about 25-30 minutes, or until the sweet potato wedges are tender and crispy, turning them once halfway through the cooking time.

7. Serve these DASH-friendly Spicy Oven-Baked Sweet Potato Wedges as a tasty and healthier alternative to traditional fries.

Nutritional Information (per serving):

- Carbs: 26g

- Fats: 7g

- Fiber: 4g

- Protein: 2g

Zesty Cucumber Radish Salad

Prep Time: 10 minutes
Cook Time: 0 minutes
Number of Servings: 4

Ingredients:

- 2 cups cucumbers, thinly sliced

- 1 cup radishes, thinly sliced

- 1/4 cup red onion, finely chopped

- 1/4 cup fresh parsley, chopped

- 2 tablespoons extra-virgin olive oil

- 1 tablespoon fresh lemon juice

- 1 teaspoon Dijon mustard

- 1/2 teaspoon honey

- 1/4 teaspoon salt

- 1/8 teaspoon black pepper

Instructions:

1. In a large mixing bowl, add the thinly sliced cucumbers, thinly sliced radishes, finely chopped red onion, and chopped fresh parsley.

2. In a separate small bowl, whisk the extra-virgin olive oil, fresh lemon juice, Dijon mustard, honey, salt, and black pepper to create the dressing.

3. Pour the dressing over the salad mixture and toss to coat the ingredients evenly.

4. Refrigerate the Zesty Cucumber Radish Salad for at least 20 minutes before serving to allow the flavors to meld.

5. Serve this DASH-friendly salad as a refreshing and crisp side dish.

Nutritional Information (per serving):

- Carbs: 6g

- Fats: 7g

- Fiber: 2g

- Protein: 1g

Smoked Salmon Cucumber Bites

Prep Time: 15 minutes
Cook Time: 0 minutes
Number of Servings: 4

Ingredients:

- 2 cucumbers, sliced into rounds
- 4 ounces smoked salmon, cut into small pieces
- 1/4 cup Greek yogurt
- 1 tablespoon fresh dill, finely chopped
- 1/2 lemon, zest and juice
- 1/4 teaspoon black pepper

Instructions:

1. In a small mixing bowl, add the Greek yogurt, finely chopped fresh dill, lemon zest, lemon juice, and black pepper. Mix sufficiently to create the dill-yogurt sauce.

2. Place the cucumber rounds on a serving platter.

3. Top each cucumber round with a small piece of smoked salmon.

4. Drizzle a small amount of the dill-yogurt sauce over each smoked salmon-topped cucumber round.

5. Serve these DASH-friendly Smoked Salmon Cucumber Bites as a delectable and nutritious appetizer or snack.

Nutritional Information (per serving):

- Carbs: 5g
- Fats: 3g
- Fiber: 1g
- Protein: 7g

Roasted Garlic and White Bean Dip

Prep Time: 10 minutes
Cook Time: 40 minutes
Number of Servings: 8

Ingredients:

- 1 whole garlic bulb

- 2 tablespoons olive oil

- 2 cans (15 ounces each) white beans (cannellini or Great Northern), drained and rinsed

- 1/4 cup fresh lemon juice

- 2 tablespoons tahini

- 1/2 teaspoon dried rosemary

- 1/4 teaspoon salt

- 1/4 teaspoon black pepper

- 1/4 teaspoon red pepper flakes (optional)

- Fresh parsley, for garnish

Instructions:

1. Preheat your oven to 400°F (200°C).

2. Cut the top off the whole garlic bulb, exposing the cloves. Place it on a piece of aluminum foil and drizzle with a tablespoon of olive oil. Wrap the garlic in the foil and roast it in the preheated oven for about 30-40 minutes, or until the garlic is soft and golden. Take out from the oven and let it cool.

3. In a food processor, add the roasted garlic cloves (squeeze the soft garlic out of the skins), drained and rinsed white beans, fresh lemon juice, tahini, dried rosemary, salt, black pepper, and red pepper

flakes if desired. Process the mixture until it is smooth and creamy, scraping down the sides of the bowl as needed.

4. Transfer the Roasted Garlic and White Bean Dip to a serving bowl and garnish with fresh parsley.

5. Serve this DASH-friendly dip with vegetable sticks, whole-grain crackers, or whole-grain pita bread.

Nutritional Information (per serving):

- Carbs: 21g

- Fats: 4g

- Fiber: 5g

- Protein: 7g

Spicy Avocado Salsa

Prep Time: 15 minutes
Cook Time: 0 minutes
Number of Servings: 4

Ingredients:

- 2 ripe avocados, diced

- 1 cup tomato, diced

- 1/4 cup red onion, finely diced

- 1/4 cup fresh cilantro, chopped

- 1 jalapeño pepper, finely diced (Take out seeds for milder salsa)

- 1/4 cup fresh lime juice

- 1/4 teaspoon salt

- 1/8 teaspoon black pepper

Instructions:

1. In a mixing bowl, add the diced ripe avocados, diced tomato, finely diced red onion, chopped fresh cilantro, and finely diced jalapeño pepper.

2. Drizzle the fresh lime juice over the mixture and gently toss to coat the ingredients.

3. Season the Spicy Avocado Salsa with salt and black pepper, and gently toss again to ensure even distribution of the seasonings.

4. Serve this DASH-friendly Spicy Avocado Salsa as a zesty and flavorful dip for tortilla chips, as a topping for grilled chicken or fish, or as a side salad.

Nutritional Information (per serving):

- Carbs: 13g

- Fats: 15g

- Fiber: 7g

- Protein: 2g

Baked Zucchini Fritters

Prep Time: 15 minutes
Cook Time: 25 minutes
Number of Servings: 4

Ingredients:

- 2 cups zucchini, grated and squeezed to remove excess moisture

- 1/4 cup whole-wheat flour

- 1/4 cup grated Parmesan cheese

- 1/4 cup fresh parsley, finely chopped

- 1/4 cup red onion, finely diced

- 1 egg

- 1/2 teaspoon garlic powder

- 1/2 teaspoon dried oregano

- 1/4 teaspoon salt

- 1/4 teaspoon black pepper

- Olive oil cooking spray

Instructions:

1. Preheat your oven to 425°F (220°C) and line a baking sheet with parchment paper. Lightly coat the parchment paper with olive oil cooking spray.

2. Grate the zucchini and place it in a clean kitchen towel or paper towels. Squeeze the zucchini to remove excess moisture.

3. In a mixing bowl, add the grated and drained zucchini, whole-wheat flour, grated Parmesan cheese, finely chopped fresh parsley, finely diced red onion, egg, garlic powder, dried oregano, salt, and black pepper. Mix sufficiently to form the fritter mixture.

4. Using a spoon, scoop out portions of the mixture and shape them into fritters. Place the fritters on the prepared baking sheet.

5. Lightly coat the tops of the fritters with olive oil cooking spray.

6. Bake in the preheated oven for about 20-25 minutes, or until the fritters are golden brown and crisp.

7. Serve these DASH-friendly Baked Zucchini Fritters as a delightful and healthier alternative to traditional fried fritters.

Nutritional Information (per serving):

- Carbs: 11g

- Fats: 6g

- Fiber: 2g

- Protein: 6g

Greek Tzatziki with Pita Bread

Prep Time: 15 minutes
Cook Time: 0 minutes
Number of Servings: 4

Ingredients:

- 1 cup Greek yogurt
- 1/2 cucumber, grated and squeezed to remove excess moisture
- 2 cloves garlic, minced
- 1 tablespoon fresh dill, finely chopped
- 1 tablespoon extra-virgin olive oil
- 1 tablespoon fresh lemon juice
- 1/4 teaspoon salt
- 1/4 teaspoon black pepper
- 4 whole-grain pita bread, for serving

Instructions:

1. In a mixing bowl, add the Greek yogurt, grated and drained cucumber, minced garlic, finely chopped fresh dill, extra-virgin olive oil, fresh lemon juice, salt, and black pepper. Mix sufficiently to create the tzatziki sauce.

2. Warm the whole-grain pita bread in a toaster or oven.

3. Serve the Greek Tzatziki with Pita Bread as a healthy and flavorful dip or sauce for the warm pita bread.

Nutritional Information (per serving):

- Carbs: 18g
- Fats: 6g
- Fiber: 4g

- Protein: 8g

Curried Lentil and Carrot Dip

Prep Time: 15 minutes
Cook Time: 25 minutes
Number of Servings: 8

Ingredients:

- 1 cup red lentils

- 3 cups water

- 2 cups carrots, peeled and diced

- 1 onion, diced

- 2 cloves garlic, minced

- 1 tablespoon olive oil

- 1 tablespoon curry powder

- 1/2 teaspoon ground cumin

- 1/4 teaspoon ground coriander

- 1/4 teaspoon ground turmeric

- 1/4 teaspoon ground cinnamon

- 1/4 teaspoon salt

- 1/8 teaspoon black pepper

- 2 tablespoons fresh cilantro, chopped

- Whole-grain pita bread or vegetable sticks, for serving

Instructions:

1. In a medium saucepan, add the red lentils and water. Bring to a boil, then reduce the heat and simmer for about 15-20 minutes, or

until the lentils are soft and most of the water is absorbed. Drain any excess water and set the cooked lentils aside.

2. In a large skillet, heat the olive oil over medium heat. Add the diced onions and cook for 2-3 minutes, or until they become translucent.

3. Add the minced garlic and diced carrots to the skillet. Sauté for an extra 5-7 minutes, or until the carrots are tender.

4. Stir in the curry powder, ground cumin, ground coriander, ground turmeric, ground cinnamon, salt, and black pepper. Cook for an additional 2-3 minutes to toast the spices.

5.   Take out the skillet from heat and let the carrot and spice mixture cool slightly.

6. In a food processor, add the cooked red lentils and the carrot and spice mixture. Process until the mixture is smooth and well blended.

7. Transfer the Curried Lentil and Carrot Dip to a serving bowl and garnish with fresh cilantro.

8. Serve this DASH-friendly dip with whole-grain pita bread or vegetable sticks as a healthy and flavorful appetizer.

Nutritional Information (per serving):

- Carbs: 25g
- Fats: 2g
- Fiber: 7g
- Protein: 9g

Teriyaki Edamame

Prep Time: 5 minutes
Cook Time: 10 minutes
Number of Servings: 4

Ingredients:

- 2 cups edamame (young soybeans), frozen and shelled
- 2 tablespoons low-sodium soy sauce
- 2 tablespoons honey
- 1 tablespoon rice vinegar
- 1/2 teaspoon ginger, grated
- 1/4 teaspoon garlic, minced
- 1/4 teaspoon sesame seeds (for garnish)
- 1 green onion, finely chopped (for garnish)

Instructions:

1. In a small bowl, whisk the low-sodium soy sauce, honey, rice vinegar, grated ginger, and minced garlic to create the teriyaki sauce.

2. In a large saucepan, bring water to a boil. Add the shelled edamame and cook for 5-7 minutes, or until tender.

3. Drain the edamame and return them to the saucepan.

4. Pour the teriyaki sauce over the cooked edamame and toss to coat them evenly. Cook for an additional 2-3 minutes to heat the sauce and caramelize it slightly.

5. Transfer the Teriyaki Edamame to a serving dish and garnish with sesame seeds and finely chopped green onions.

6. Serve this DASH-friendly Teriyaki Edamame as a delicious and nutritious appetizer or snack.

Nutritional Information (per serving):

- Carbs: 19g
- Fats: 2g

- Fiber: 4g

- Protein: 9g

Beet and Goat Cheese Crostini

Prep Time: 15 minutes
Cook Time: 0 minutes
Number of Servings: 4

Ingredients:

- 4 slices whole-grain baguette or French bread

- 4 ounces goat cheese

- 2 small beets, cooked, peeled, and sliced

- 1/4 cup fresh arugula

- 1/4 cup balsamic glaze

- 1/4 teaspoon black pepper

- 1/8 teaspoon salt

- 1/8 teaspoon olive oil

Instructions:

1. Preheat your oven's broiler.

2. Lightly brush the slices of whole-grain baguette or French bread with olive oil. Place them on a baking sheet and toast them under the broiler for about 1-2 minutes on each side, or until they are golden brown and crispy.

3. Spread goat cheese evenly on each toasted bread slice.

4. Top the goat cheese with sliced cooked beets.

5. In a small mixing bowl, toss fresh arugula with a pinch of salt and black pepper.

6. Place a small handful of seasoned arugula on top of the beets on each crostini.

7. Drizzle balsamic glaze over the Beet and Goat Cheese Crostini.

8. Serve these DASH-friendly crostini as a delightful and elegant appetizer.

Nutritional Information (per serving):

- Carbs: 24g

- Fats: 7g

- Fiber: 4g

- Protein: 10g

Chapter 5: Soups & Stews

Minestrone Soup Recipe

Prep Time: 20 minutes
Cook Time: 30 minutes
Number of Servings: 6

Ingredients:

- 2 cups low-sodium vegetable broth

- 1 cup water

- 1 can (14.5 oz) no-salt-added diced tomatoes

- 1 cup chopped carrots, diced

- 1 cup chopped celery, diced

- 1 cup diced zucchini

- 1 cup diced green beans

- 1 cup chopped onion, diced

- 2 cloves garlic, minced

- 1 teaspoon dried basil

- 1 teaspoon dried oregano

- 1/2 teaspoon salt

- 1/4 teaspoon black pepper

- 1 can (15 oz) low-sodium kidney beans, drained and rinsed

- 1 cup whole wheat pasta (small shells or elbow macaroni)

- 1 cup chopped spinach

- 2 tablespoons grated Parmesan cheese (optional)

Instructions:

1. In a large pot, add the low-sodium vegetable broth and water. Bring to a boil over medium-high heat.

2. Add the diced tomatoes, chopped carrots, diced celery, diced zucchini, diced green beans, diced onion, minced garlic, dried basil, dried oregano, salt, and black pepper. Stir sufficiently.

3. Reduce the heat to low and let the soup simmer for about 20 minutes, or until the vegetables are tender.

4. Add the low-sodium kidney beans and whole wheat pasta. Continue to simmer for an additional 10 minutes, or until the pasta is cooked al dente.

5. Just before serving, stir in the chopped spinach and cook until wilted, which should only take a couple of minutes.

6. Ladle the DASH-friendly Minestrone Soup into bowls. If desired, top each serving with one teaspoon of grated Parmesan cheese.

Nutritional Information (per serving):

- Carbs: 38g

- Fats: 1.5g

- Fiber: 7g

- Protein: 6g

Lentil and Vegetable Soup Recipe

Prep Time: 15 minutes
Cook Time: 40 minutes
Number of Servings: 6

Ingredients:

- 2 cups low-sodium vegetable broth

- 1 cup water

- 1 cup dried green or brown lentils

- 1 cup chopped carrots, diced
- 1 cup chopped celery, diced
- 1 cup chopped onion, diced
- 2 cloves garlic, minced
- 1 can (14.5 oz) no-salt-added diced tomatoes
- 1 teaspoon dried thyme
- 1/2 teaspoon salt
- 1/4 teaspoon black pepper
- 2 cups chopped kale, stems Take outd
- 1 tablespoon olive oil
- 2 tablespoons lemon juice

Instructions:

1. In a large pot, add the low-sodium vegetable broth and water. Bring it to a boil over medium-high heat.

2. Add the dried lentils, chopped carrots, diced celery, diced onion, and minced garlic to the pot. Stir sufficiently.

3. Reduce the heat to low and let the soup simmer for about 30 minutes, or until the lentils and vegetables are tender.

4. Stir in the no-salt-added diced tomatoes, dried thyme, salt, and black pepper. Continue to simmer for an additional 10 minutes.

5. In a separate pan, heat the olive oil over medium heat. Add the chopped kale and sauté until it wilts, which should take about 5 minutes.

6. Add the sautéed kale to the soup and stir in the lemon juice. Cook for an additional 5 minutes, allowing the flavors to blend.

7. Serve the DASH-friendly Lentil and Vegetable Soup hot.

Nutritional Information (per serving):

- Carbs: 36g

- Fats: 2.5g

- Fiber: 8g

- Protein: 9g

Chicken and Rice Soup Recipe

Prep Time: 15 minutes
Cook Time: 45 minutes
Number of Servings: 6

Ingredients:

- 2 cups low-sodium chicken broth

- 2 cups water

- 1 cup brown rice

- 1 cup diced carrots

- 1 cup diced celery

- 1 cup chopped onion

- 2 cloves garlic, minced

- 1 cup cooked chicken breast, diced

- 1 teaspoon dried thyme

- 1/2 teaspoon salt

- 1/4 teaspoon black pepper

- 1 cup chopped spinach

- 2 tablespoons olive oil

- 2 tablespoons lemon juice

Instructions:

1. In a large pot, add the low-sodium chicken broth and water. Bring it to a boil over medium-high heat.

2. Add the brown rice, diced carrots, diced celery, chopped onion, and minced garlic to the pot. Stir sufficiently.

3. Reduce the heat to low, cover, and let the soup simmer for about 30 minutes, or until the rice and vegetables are tender.

4. Stir in the diced cooked chicken breast, dried thyme, salt, and black pepper. Continue to simmer for an additional 10 minutes.

5. In a separate pan, heat the olive oil over medium heat. Add the chopped spinach and sauté until it wilts, which should take about 5 minutes.

6. Add the sautéed spinach to the soup and stir in the lemon juice. Cook for an additional 5 minutes, allowing the flavors to blend.

7. Serve the DASH-friendly Chicken and Rice Soup hot.

Nutritional Information (per serving):

- Carbs: 32g

- Fats: 5g

- Fiber: 3g

- Protein: 10g

Tomato Basil Soup Recipe

Prep Time: 15 minutes
Cook Time: 25 minutes
Number of Servings: 4

Ingredients:

- 2 cups low-sodium tomato juice

- 1 cup low-sodium vegetable broth

- 1 cup diced tomatoes

- 1/2 cup chopped onion

- 2 cloves garlic, minced

- 1/4 cup chopped fresh basil leaves

- 1/2 teaspoon dried oregano

- 1/4 teaspoon salt

- 1/4 teaspoon black pepper

- 1/4 cup low-fat plain yogurt (optional, for garnish)

Instructions:

1. In a large pot, add the low-sodium tomato juice and low-sodium vegetable broth. Bring it to a boil over medium-high heat.

2. Add the diced tomatoes, chopped onion, minced garlic, chopped fresh basil leaves, dried oregano, salt, and black pepper to the pot. Stir sufficiently.

3. Reduce the heat to low and let the soup simmer for about 20 minutes, allowing the flavors to meld.

4. Use an immersion blender to puree the soup until smooth. Alternatively, transfer the soup in batches to a blender and puree until smooth, then return it to the pot.

5. Serve the DASH-friendly Tomato Basil Soup hot. If desired, top each serving with one tablespoon of low-fat plain yogurt for a creamy garnish.

Nutritional Information (per serving):

- Carbs: 15g

- Fats: 1g

- Fiber: 3g

- Protein: 2g

Spinach and White Bean Soup Recipe

Prep Time: 15 minutes
Cook Time: 25 minutes
Number of Servings: 6

Ingredients:

- 4 cups low-sodium vegetable broth
- 2 cups water
- 2 cups chopped fresh spinach
- 1 cup diced carrots
- 1 cup diced celery
- 1 cup chopped onion
- 3 cloves garlic, minced
- 2 cans (15 oz each) low-sodium white beans, drained and rinsed
- 1 teaspoon dried thyme
- 1/2 teaspoon salt
- 1/4 teaspoon black pepper
- 2 tablespoons olive oil
- 2 tablespoons lemon juice

Instructions:

1. In a large pot, add the low-sodium vegetable broth and water. Bring it to a boil over medium-high heat.

2. Add the chopped fresh spinach, diced carrots, diced celery, chopped onion, and minced garlic to the pot. Stir sufficiently.

3. Reduce the heat to low and let the soup simmer for about 20 minutes, or until the vegetables are tender.

4. Stir in the low-sodium white beans, dried thyme, salt, and black pepper. Continue to simmer for an additional 5 minutes, allowing the flavors to meld.

5. In a separate pan, heat the olive oil over medium heat. Add the lemon juice and sauté for a minute.

6. Add the sautéed olive oil and lemon juice mixture to the soup, stirring well.

7. Serve the DASH-friendly Spinach and White Bean Soup hot.

Nutritional Information (per serving):

- Carbs: 29g

- Fats: 4g

- Fiber: 7g

- Protein: 8g

Turkey and Quinoa Stew Recipe

Prep Time: 15 minutes
Cook Time: 35 minutes
Number of Servings: 4

Ingredients:

- 2 cups low-sodium chicken broth

- 1 cup water

- 1 cup diced turkey breast

- 1/2 cup quinoa, rinsed and drained

- 1 cup diced carrots

- 1 cup diced celery

- 1 cup chopped onion

- 2 cloves garlic, minced

- 1 teaspoon dried thyme

- 1/2 teaspoon salt

- 1/4 teaspoon black pepper

- 1 cup chopped kale, stems Take outd

- 2 tablespoons lemon juice

Instructions:

1. In a large pot, add the low-sodium chicken broth and water. Bring it to a boil over medium-high heat.

2. Add the diced turkey breast, rinsed and drained quinoa, diced carrots, diced celery, chopped onion, minced garlic, dried thyme, salt, and black pepper to the pot. Stir sufficiently.

3. Reduce the heat to low and let the stew simmer for about 25 minutes, or until the turkey is cooked through, quinoa is tender, and vegetables are soft.

4. Stir in the chopped kale and continue to simmer for an additional 5 minutes, allowing the kale to wilt.

5. Just before serving, add the lemon juice to the stew and mix sufficiently.

6. Serve the DASH-friendly Turkey and Quinoa Stew hot.

Nutritional Information (per serving):

- Carbs: 30g

- Fats: 2g

- Fiber: 5g

- Protein: 20g

Butternut Squash and Carrot Soup Recipe

Prep Time: 15 minutes
Cook Time: 40 minutes
Number of Servings: 6

Ingredients:

- 4 cups low-sodium vegetable broth
- 2 cups diced butternut squash
- 1 cup diced carrots
- 1 cup chopped onion
- 2 cloves garlic, minced
- 1 teaspoon dried thyme
- 1/2 teaspoon salt
- 1/4 teaspoon black pepper
- 1/2 cup low-fat plain yogurt (optional, for garnish)

Instructions:

1. In a large pot, add the low-sodium vegetable broth, diced butternut squash, diced carrots, chopped onion, minced garlic, dried thyme, salt, and black pepper.

2. Bring the mixture to a boil over medium-high heat.

3. Reduce the heat to low and let the soup simmer for about 30 minutes, or until the butternut squash and carrots are tender.

4. Use an immersion blender to puree the soup until smooth. Alternatively, transfer the soup in batches to a blender and puree until smooth, then return it to the pot.

5. Serve the DASH-friendly Butternut Squash and Carrot Soup hot. If desired, top each serving with one tablespoon of low-fat plain yogurt for a creamy garnish.

Nutritional Information (per serving):

- Carbs: 20g

- Fats: 0.5g

- Fiber: 4g

- Protein: 2g

Black Bean and Vegetable Stew Recipe

Prep Time: 20 minutes
Cook Time: 30 minutes
Number of Servings: 6

Ingredients:

- 2 cups low-sodium vegetable broth

- 1 cup water

- 2 cans (15 oz each) low-sodium black beans, drained and rinsed

- 1 cup diced carrots

- 1 cup diced celery

- 1 cup chopped onion

- 2 cloves garlic, minced

- 1 cup diced zucchini

- 1 cup diced bell peppers (any color)

- 1 teaspoon dried cumin

- 1/2 teaspoon salt

- 1/4 teaspoon black pepper

- 1/4 cup chopped fresh cilantro

- 1 tablespoon olive oil

Instructions:

1. In a large pot, add the low-sodium vegetable broth and water. Bring it to a boil over medium-high heat.

2. Add the drained and rinsed low-sodium black beans, diced carrots, diced celery, chopped onion, minced garlic, diced zucchini, diced bell peppers, dried cumin, salt, and black pepper to the pot. Stir sufficiently.

3. Reduce the heat to low and let the stew simmer for about 20 minutes, allowing the vegetables to become tender.

4. In a separate pan, heat the olive oil over medium heat. Sauté the fresh cilantro for a minute.

5. Add the sautéed cilantro to the stew and let it simmer for an additional 10 minutes to meld the flavors.

6. Serve the DASH-friendly Black Bean and Vegetable Stew hot.

Nutritional Information (per serving):

- Carbs: 29g
- Fats: 3g
- Fiber: 8g
- Protein: 9g

Moroccan Lentil Soup Recipe

Prep Time: 20 minutes
Cook Time: 40 minutes
Number of Servings: 6

Ingredients:

- 4 cups low-sodium vegetable broth
- 2 cups water

- 1 cup dried red lentils
- 1 cup diced carrots
- 1 cup chopped onion
- 1 cup diced celery
- 2 cloves garlic, minced
- 1 can (14.5 oz) no-salt-added diced tomatoes
- 1 teaspoon ground cumin
- 1/2 teaspoon ground coriander
- 1/2 teaspoon ground cinnamon
- 1/4 teaspoon ground turmeric
- 1/2 teaspoon salt
- 1/4 teaspoon black pepper
- 2 tablespoons olive oil
- 2 tablespoons lemon juice

Instructions:

1. In a large pot, add the low-sodium vegetable broth and water. Bring it to a boil over medium-high heat.

2. Add the dried red lentils, diced carrots, chopped onion, diced celery, minced garlic, and no-salt-added diced tomatoes to the pot. Stir sufficiently.

3. Season the mixture with ground cumin, ground coriander, ground cinnamon, ground turmeric, salt, and black pepper.

4. Reduce the heat to low and let the soup simmer for about 30 minutes, or until the lentils and vegetables are tender.

5. In a separate pan, heat the olive oil over medium heat. Add the lemon juice and sauté for a minute.

6. Add the sautéed olive oil and lemon juice mixture to the soup, stirring well.

7. Serve the DASH-friendly Moroccan Lentil Soup hot.

Nutritional Information (per serving):

- Carbs: 26g

- Fats: 5g

- Fiber: 7g

- Protein: 9g

Creamy Broccoli and Potato Soup Recipe

Prep Time: 20 minutes
Cook Time: 30 minutes
Number of Servings: 4

Ingredients:

- 4 cups low-sodium vegetable broth

- 2 cups water

- 2 cups diced potatoes

- 2 cups chopped broccoli florets

- 1 cup chopped onion

- 2 cloves garlic, minced

- 1/2 cup low-fat plain yogurt

- 1/2 cup low-fat milk

- 1/2 teaspoon dried thyme

- 1/2 teaspoon salt

- 1/4 teaspoon black pepper

Instructions:

1. In a large pot, add the low-sodium vegetable broth and water. Bring it to a boil over medium-high heat.

2. Add the diced potatoes, chopped broccoli florets, chopped onion, and minced garlic to the pot. Stir sufficiently.

3. Reduce the heat to low and let the soup simmer for about 20 minutes, or until the potatoes and broccoli are tender.

4. Use an immersion blender to puree the soup until smooth. Alternatively, transfer the soup in batches to a blender and puree until smooth, then return it to the pot.

5. Stir in the low-fat plain yogurt, low-fat milk, dried thyme, salt, and black pepper. Continue to cook for an additional 10 minutes, allowing the flavors to meld.

6. Serve the DASH-friendly Creamy Broccoli and Potato Soup hot.

Nutritional Information (per serving):

- Carbs: 30g
- Fats: 1.5g
- Fiber: 4g
- Protein: 6g

Cabbage and Sausage Stew Recipe

Prep Time: 20 minutes
Cook Time: 40 minutes
Number of Servings: 6

Ingredients:

- 4 cups low-sodium chicken broth
- 2 cups water

- 2 cups diced cabbage

- 1 cup diced carrots

- 1 cup diced onion

- 1 cup diced celery

- 1 cup chopped bell peppers (any color)

- 2 cloves garlic, minced

- 12 ounces low-sodium turkey or chicken sausage, sliced

- 1 teaspoon dried thyme

- 1/2 teaspoon salt

- 1/4 teaspoon black pepper

Instructions:

1. In a large pot, add the low-sodium chicken broth and water. Bring it to a boil over medium-high heat.

2. Add the diced cabbage, diced carrots, diced onion, diced celery, chopped bell peppers, and minced garlic to the pot. Stir sufficiently.

3. In a separate pan, brown the sliced low-sodium turkey or chicken sausage until it's cooked through. Drain any excess fat.

4. Add the cooked sausage to the pot with the vegetables.

5. Season the stew with dried thyme, salt, and black pepper.

6. Reduce the heat to low and let the stew simmer for about 30 minutes, allowing the flavors to meld.

7. Serve the DASH-friendly Cabbage and Sausage Stew hot.

Nutritional Information (per serving):

- Carbs: 18g

- Fats: 6g

- Fiber: 4g

- Protein: 14g

Mushroom Barley Soup Recipe

Prep Time: 20 minutes
Cook Time: 45 minutes
Number of Servings: 6

Ingredients:

- 6 cups low-sodium vegetable broth

- 1 cup water

- 1 cup pearl barley

- 2 cups sliced mushrooms

- 1 cup diced carrots

- 1 cup diced celery

- 1 cup chopped onion

- 2 cloves garlic, minced

- 1 teaspoon dried thyme

- 1/2 teaspoon salt

- 1/4 teaspoon black pepper

Instructions:

1. In a large pot, add the low-sodium vegetable broth and water. Bring it to a boil over medium-high heat.

2. Add the pearl barley, sliced mushrooms, diced carrots, diced celery, chopped onion, minced garlic, dried thyme, salt, and black pepper to the pot. Stir sufficiently.

3. Reduce the heat to low and let the soup simmer for about 40 minutes, or until the barley and vegetables are tender.

4. Serve the DASH-friendly Mushroom Barley Soup hot.

Nutritional Information (per serving):

- Carbs: 34g
- Fats: 1.5g
- Fiber: 6g
- Protein: 4g

Thai Red Curry Soup Recipe

Prep Time: 15 minutes
Cook Time: 25 minutes
Number of Servings: 4

Ingredients:

- 4 cups low-sodium vegetable broth
- 1 cup water
- 1 cup diced tofu
- 1 cup diced red bell pepper
- 1 cup sliced mushrooms
- 1/2 cup diced carrots
- 1/2 cup diced zucchini
- 1/2 cup chopped onion
- 2 cloves garlic, minced
- 2 tablespoons Thai red curry paste
- 1/2 teaspoon salt
- 1/4 teaspoon black pepper
- 1/2 cup light coconut milk

- 1 tablespoon fresh cilantro, chopped

- 1 tablespoon fresh basil, chopped

Instructions:

1. In a large pot, add the low-sodium vegetable broth and water. Bring it to a boil over medium-high heat.

2. Add the diced tofu, diced red bell pepper, sliced mushrooms, diced carrots, diced zucchini, chopped onion, minced garlic, Thai red curry paste, salt, and black pepper to the pot. Stir sufficiently.

3. Reduce the heat to low and let the soup simmer for about 20 minutes, allowing the vegetables to become tender.

4. Stir in the light coconut milk and cook for an additional 5 minutes, letting the flavors blend.

5. Serve the DASH-friendly Thai Red Curry Soup hot. Garnish each serving with chopped fresh cilantro and basil.

Nutritional Information (per serving):

- Carbs: 15g

- Fats: 7g

- Fiber: 3g

- Protein: 7g

Mexican Chicken and Vegetable Soup Recipe

Prep Time: 20 minutes
Cook Time: 35 minutes
Number of Servings: 6

Ingredients:

- 4 cups low-sodium chicken broth

- 2 cups water

- 1 cup diced chicken breast

- 1 cup diced bell peppers (any color)

- 1 cup diced zucchini

- 1 cup chopped onion

- 2 cloves garlic, minced

- 1 cup no-salt-added corn kernels

- 1 can (15 oz) no-salt-added black beans, drained and rinsed

- 1 teaspoon ground cumin

- 1/2 teaspoon chili powder

- 1/2 teaspoon salt

- 1/4 teaspoon black pepper

- 1/4 cup low-fat plain yogurt (optional, for garnish)

Instructions:

1. In a large pot, add the low-sodium chicken broth and water. Bring it to a boil over medium-high heat.

2. Add the diced chicken breast, diced bell peppers, diced zucchini, chopped onion, minced garlic, no-salt-added corn kernels, and drained and rinsed no-salt-added black beans to the pot. Stir sufficiently.

3. Season the soup with ground cumin, chili powder, salt, and black pepper.

4. Reduce the heat to low and let the soup simmer for about 30 minutes, allowing the vegetables to become tender.

5. Serve the DASH-friendly Mexican Chicken and Vegetable Soup hot. If desired, top each serving with one tablespoon of low-fat plain yogurt for a creamy garnish.

Nutritional Information (per serving):

- Carbs: 23g

- Fats: 2g

- Fiber: 6g

- Protein: 13g

Sweet Potato and Lentil Soup Recipe

Prep Time: 15 minutes
Cook Time: 35 minutes
Number of Servings: 6

Ingredients:

- 4 cups low-sodium vegetable broth

- 2 cups water

- 2 cups diced sweet potatoes

- 1 cup dried red lentils

- 1 cup chopped onion

- 2 cloves garlic, minced

- 1 teaspoon ground cumin

- 1/2 teaspoon ground coriander

- 1/2 teaspoon ground cinnamon

- 1/4 teaspoon ground turmeric

- 1/2 teaspoon salt

- 1/4 teaspoon black pepper

- 1/4 cup plain Greek yogurt (optional, for garnish)

Instructions:

1. In a large pot, add the low-sodium vegetable broth and water. Bring it to a boil over medium-high heat.

2. Add the diced sweet potatoes, dried red lentils, chopped onion, minced garlic, ground cumin, ground coriander, ground cinnamon, ground turmeric, salt, and black pepper to the pot. Stir sufficiently.

3. Reduce the heat to low and let the soup simmer for about 30 minutes, or until the sweet potatoes and lentils are tender.

4. Use an immersion blender to puree the soup until smooth. Alternatively, transfer the soup in batches to a blender and puree until smooth, then return it to the pot.

5. Serve the DASH-friendly Sweet Potato and Lentil Soup hot. If desired, top each serving with one tablespoon of plain Greek yogurt for a creamy garnish.

Nutritional Information (per serving):

- Carbs: 30g

- Fats: 1g

- Fiber: 10g

- Protein: 9g

Chicken and Vegetable Quinoa Soup Recipe

Prep Time: 20 minutes
Cook Time: 35 minutes
Number of Servings: 6

Ingredients:

- 4 cups low-sodium chicken broth

- 2 cups water

- 1 cup cooked and diced chicken breast

- 1 cup diced carrots

- 1 cup diced celery

- 1 cup chopped onion
- 1 cup chopped bell peppers (any color)
- 1 cup diced zucchini
- 1/2 cup quinoa, rinsed and drained
- 2 cloves garlic, minced
- 1 teaspoon dried thyme
- 1/2 teaspoon salt
- 1/4 teaspoon black pepper

Instructions:

1. In a large pot, add the low-sodium chicken broth and water. Bring it to a boil over medium-high heat.

2. Add the cooked and diced chicken breast, diced carrots, diced celery, chopped onion, chopped bell peppers, diced zucchini, quinoa (rinsed and drained), minced garlic, dried thyme, salt, and black pepper to the pot. Stir sufficiently.

3. Reduce the heat to low and let the soup simmer for about 30 minutes, or until the quinoa and vegetables are tender.

4. Serve the DASH-friendly Chicken and Vegetable Quinoa Soup hot.

Nutritional Information (per serving):

- Carbs: 21g
- Fats: 2.5g
- Fiber: 4g
- Protein: 14g

Italian Wedding Soup Recipe

Prep Time: 30 minutes
Cook Time: 45 minutes
Number of Servings: 6

Ingredients:

- 6 cups low-sodium chicken broth

- 2 cups water

- 1 cup lean ground turkey

- 1/2 cup whole wheat breadcrumbs

- 1/4 cup grated Parmesan cheese

- 1/4 cup chopped fresh parsley

- 1/2 cup diced carrots

- 1/2 cup chopped spinach

- 1/2 cup diced onion

- 2 cloves garlic, minced

- 1 cup small pasta (e.g., orzo or ditalini)

- 1/2 teaspoon salt

- 1/4 teaspoon black pepper

Instructions:

1. In a large pot, add the low-sodium chicken broth and water. Bring it to a boil over medium-high heat.

2. In a mixing bowl, add the lean ground turkey, whole wheat breadcrumbs, grated Parmesan cheese, and chopped fresh parsley. Roll into small meatballs, about 1 inch in diameter.

3. Add the meatballs, diced carrots, chopped spinach, diced onion, minced garlic, small pasta, salt, and black pepper to the pot. Stir sufficiently.

4. Reduce the heat to low and let the soup simmer for about 30 minutes, allowing the meatballs to cook through and the pasta to become tender.

5. Serve the DASH-friendly Italian Wedding Soup hot.

Nutritional Information (per serving):

- Carbs: 18g

- Fats: 4g

- Fiber: 2g

- Protein: 14g

Creamy Spinach and Potato Soup Recipe

Prep Time: 20 minutes
Cook Time: 35 minutes
Number of Servings: 6

Ingredients:

- 4 cups low-sodium vegetable broth

- 2 cups water

- 2 cups diced potatoes

- 1 cup chopped onion

- 2 cloves garlic, minced

- 4 cups fresh spinach, chopped

- 1 cup low-fat milk

- 2 tablespoons whole wheat flour

- 1/2 teaspoon dried thyme

- 1/2 teaspoon salt

- 1/4 teaspoon black pepper

Instructions:

1. In a large pot, add the low-sodium vegetable broth and water. Bring it to a boil over medium-high heat.

2. Add the diced potatoes, chopped onion, and minced garlic to the pot. Stir sufficiently.

3. Reduce the heat to low and let the soup simmer for about 20 minutes, or until the potatoes are tender.

4. In a separate bowl, whisk the low-fat milk and whole wheat flour until smooth.

5. Slowly pour the milk and flour mixture into the soup, stirring continuously.

6. Add the chopped fresh spinach, dried thyme, salt, and black pepper to the pot. Continue to cook for an additional 10 minutes, allowing the flavors to meld and the soup to thicken.

7. Serve the DASH-friendly Creamy Spinach and Potato Soup hot.

Nutritional Information (per serving):

- Carbs: 20g
- Fats: 1g
- Fiber: 3g
- Protein: 3g

Lemon Herb Shrimp and Vegetable Stew Recipe

Prep Time: 20 minutes
Cook Time: 25 minutes
Number of Servings: 4

Ingredients:

- 4 cups low-sodium vegetable broth

- 2 cups water

- 1 pound large shrimp, peeled and deveined

- 2 cups diced zucchini

- 1 cup diced carrots

- 1 cup diced celery

- 1 cup chopped onion

- 2 cloves garlic, minced

- 1 lemon, zested and juiced

- 1/4 cup fresh parsley, chopped

- 1/2 teaspoon dried thyme

- 1/2 teaspoon salt

- 1/4 teaspoon black pepper

- 1 tablespoon olive oil

Instructions:

1. In a large pot, add the low-sodium vegetable broth and water. Bring it to a boil over medium-high heat.

2. Add the diced zucchini, diced carrots, diced celery, chopped onion, and minced garlic to the pot. Stir sufficiently.

3. Season the soup with dried thyme, salt, and black pepper.

4. Reduce the heat to low and let the soup simmer for about 20 minutes, allowing the vegetables to become tender.

5. In a separate pan, heat the olive oil over medium heat. Add the peeled and deveined large shrimp, lemon zest, and lemon juice. Sauté until the shrimp turn pink and are cooked through, about 3-4 minutes.

6. Add the cooked shrimp and fresh parsley to the soup. Stir to combine.

7. Serve the DASH-friendly Lemon Herb Shrimp and Vegetable Stew hot.

Nutritional Information (per serving):

- Carbs: 12g

- Fats: 3.5g

- Fiber: 3g

- Protein: 21g

Thai Coconut Curry Chicken Soup Recipe

Prep Time: 15 minutes
Cook Time: 25 minutes
Number of Servings: 4

Ingredients:

- 4 cups low-sodium chicken broth

- 2 cups water

- 1 pound boneless, skinless chicken breast, thinly sliced

- 1 cup sliced mushrooms

- 1 cup sliced red bell pepper

- 1 cup chopped bok choy

- 1/2 cup sliced carrots

- 1/2 cup diced onion

- 2 cloves garlic, minced

- 1 can (13.5 oz) light coconut milk

- 2 tablespoons Thai red curry paste

- 1 tablespoon fish sauce

- 1 teaspoon brown sugar

- 1/2 teaspoon salt

- 1/4 teaspoon black pepper

- 1 tablespoon fresh cilantro, chopped (for garnish)

- 1 tablespoon fresh basil, chopped (for garnish)

Instructions:

1. In a large pot, add the low-sodium chicken broth and water. Bring it to a boil over medium-high heat.

2. Add the thinly sliced boneless, skinless chicken breast, sliced mushrooms, sliced red bell pepper, chopped bok choy, sliced carrots, diced onion, and minced garlic to the pot. Stir sufficiently.

3. In a separate bowl, whisk the light coconut milk, Thai red curry paste, fish sauce, brown sugar, salt, and black pepper.

4. Pour the coconut milk mixture into the pot and stir to combine.

5. Reduce the heat to low and let the soup simmer for about 20 minutes, allowing the chicken to cook through and the vegetables to become tender.

6. Serve the DASH-friendly Thai Coconut Curry Chicken Soup hot. Garnish each serving with chopped fresh cilantro and basil.

Nutritional Information (per serving):

- Carbs: 15g

- Fats: 7g

- Fiber: 3g

- Protein: 27g

Red Lentil and Spinach Stew Recipe

Prep Time: 15 minutes
Cook Time: 30 minutes
Number of Servings: 6

Ingredients:

- 4 cups low-sodium vegetable broth
- 2 cups water
- 1 cup dried red lentils
- 1 cup diced carrots
- 1 cup diced celery
- 1 cup diced onion
- 2 cloves garlic, minced
- 4 cups fresh spinach, chopped
- 1 teaspoon ground cumin
- 1/2 teaspoon ground coriander
- 1/2 teaspoon ground turmeric
- 1/2 teaspoon salt
- 1/4 teaspoon black pepper

Instructions:

1. In a large pot, add the low-sodium vegetable broth and water. Bring it to a boil over medium-high heat.

2. Add the dried red lentils, diced carrots, diced celery, diced onion, and minced garlic to the pot. Stir sufficiently.

3. Season the stew with ground cumin, ground coriander, ground turmeric, salt, and black pepper.

4. Reduce the heat to low and let the stew simmer for about 25 minutes, or until the lentils and vegetables are tender.

5. Stir in the chopped fresh spinach and let it cook for an additional 5 minutes, allowing the spinach to wilt.

6. Serve the DASH-friendly Red Lentil and Spinach Stew hot.

Nutritional Information (per serving):

- Carbs: 24g

- Fats: 1g

- Fiber: 8g

- Protein: 9g

Chapter 6: Main Courses

Grilled Lemon Herb Chicken

Prep Time: 15 minutes
Cook Time: 20 minutes
Number of Servings: 4

Ingredients:

- 4 boneless, skinless chicken breasts (about 1.5 pounds)
- 2 lemons, zested and juiced
- 2 tablespoons olive oil
- 1 teaspoon dried oregano
- 1 teaspoon dried thyme
- 1 teaspoon dried rosemary
- 1/2 teaspoon garlic powder
- 1/2 teaspoon onion powder
- Salt and pepper to taste
- 2 tablespoons fresh parsley, finely chopped

Instructions:

1. In a small bowl, add the lemon zest, lemon juice, olive oil, dried oregano, dried thyme, dried rosemary, garlic powder, onion powder, salt, and pepper. This will be your marinade.

2. Place the chicken breasts in a large resealable plastic bag or a shallow dish. Pour the marinade over the chicken, ensuring it's well coated. Seal the bag or cover the dish and refrigerate for at least 1 hour, or ideally, marinate overnight.

3. Preheat your grill to medium-high heat (about 400°F or 200°C).

4. Take out the chicken from the marinade and let any excess drip off.

5. Grill the chicken for about 6-8 minutes per side, or until the internal temperature reaches 165°F (74°C) and the chicken is no longer pink in the center.

6. While grilling, you can baste the chicken with the remaining marinade for extra flavor.

7. Once cooked, take out the chicken from the grill and let it rest for a few minutes.

8. Sprinkle the grilled chicken with freshly chopped parsley before serving.

Nutritional Information (Per Serving):

- Carbs: 5 grams

- Fats: 9 grams

- Fiber: 1 gram

- Protein: 30 grams

Baked Salmon with Dill Sauce

Prep Time: 10 minutes
Cook Time: 15 minutes
Number of Servings: 4

Ingredients:

- 4 salmon fillets (about 1.5 pounds)

- 2 tablespoons fresh dill, finely chopped

- 2 tablespoons Dijon mustard

- 2 tablespoons olive oil

- 2 tablespoons lemon juice

- 1 teaspoon garlic powder

- 1/2 teaspoon black pepper

- 1/4 teaspoon salt

- 1 lemon, thinly sliced

- 2 teaspoons capers (optional)

Instructions:

1. Preheat your oven to 375°F (190°C).

2. In a small bowl, add the fresh dill, Dijon mustard, olive oil, lemon juice, garlic powder, black pepper, and salt to create the dill sauce.

3. Place the salmon fillets on a baking sheet lined with parchment paper or lightly greased.

4. Spread a generous portion of the dill sauce evenly over each salmon fillet.

5. Place a couple of lemon slices on top of each fillet, and add capers if desired.

6. Bake the salmon in the preheated oven for approximately 15 minutes or until the salmon easily flakes with a fork.

7. Once baked, take out the salmon from the oven.

8. Serve the baked salmon with additional dill sauce on the side.

Nutritional Information (Per Serving):

- Carbs: 3 grams

- Fats: 17 grams

- Fiber: 1 gram

- Protein: 29 grams

Black Bean and Sweet Potato Tacos

Prep Time: 15 minutes
Cook Time: 30 minutes
Number of Servings: 4

Ingredients:

- 2 cups sweet potatoes, peeled and diced
- 1 can (15 ounces) black beans, drained and rinsed
- 1 tablespoon olive oil
- 1 teaspoon chili powder
- 1/2 teaspoon cumin
- 1/2 teaspoon paprika
- 1/4 teaspoon garlic powder
- 1/4 teaspoon onion powder
- Salt and pepper to taste
- 8 small whole-wheat tortillas
- 1 cup shredded lettuce
- 1 cup diced tomatoes
- 1/2 cup diced red onion
- 1/2 cup plain Greek yogurt (non-fat)
- 1/4 cup fresh cilantro, chopped
- 1 lime, cut into wedges

Instructions:

1. In a mixing bowl, add the diced sweet potatoes, olive oil, chili powder, cumin, paprika, garlic powder, onion powder, salt, and pepper. Toss until the sweet potatoes are well coated with the seasoning.

2. Spread the seasoned sweet potatoes on a baking sheet and roast in a preheated oven at 425°F (220°C) for about 25-30 minutes or until they are tender and slightly crispy.

3. While the sweet potatoes are roasting, warm the black beans in a saucepan over low heat. Season with a pinch of salt, pepper, and a dash of cumin. Keep warm until ready to use.

4. Warm the whole-wheat tortillas in a dry skillet or microwave according to the package instructions.

5. Assemble the tacos by placing a scoop of roasted sweet potatoes on each tortilla, followed by black beans, shredded lettuce, diced tomatoes, and diced red onion.

6. Drizzle each taco with a dollop of plain Greek yogurt and sprinkle with fresh cilantro.

7. Serve the tacos with lime wedges for a burst of fresh citrus flavor.

Nutritional Information (Per Serving):

- Carbs: 47 grams

- Fats: 7 grams

- Fiber: 10 grams

- Protein: 13 grams

Spaghetti Squash with Pesto

Prep Time: 10 minutes
Cook Time: 40 minutes
Number of Servings: 4

Ingredients:

- 1 medium-sized spaghetti squash

- 2 cups fresh basil leaves

- 1/4 cup pine nuts

- 1/4 cup grated Parmesan cheese

- 2 cloves garlic, minced

- 1/4 cup extra-virgin olive oil

- Salt and pepper to taste

- 1/4 cup cherry tomatoes, halved (for garnish, optional)

Instructions:

1. Preheat your oven to 375°F (190°C).

2. Cut the spaghetti squash in half lengthwise and scoop out the seeds and stringy bits.

3. Place the squash halves, cut side down, on a baking sheet. Roast in the preheated oven for about 30-40 minutes or until the squash is tender when pierced with a fork. Take out from the oven and let it cool for a few minutes.

4. While the squash is cooling, prepare the pesto. In a food processor, add the basil leaves, pine nuts, grated Parmesan cheese, minced garlic, and a pinch of salt and pepper. Pulse the ingredients until they are finely chopped.

5. With the food processor running, slowly drizzle in the extra-virgin olive oil until the pesto is well combined. Taste and adjust the salt and pepper if needed.

6. Using a fork, scrape the flesh of the roasted spaghetti squash into spaghetti-like strands. Place the strands in a serving bowl.

7. Add the prepared pesto to the spaghetti squash strands and toss to coat them evenly.

8. If desired, garnish the dish with halved cherry tomatoes.

Nutritional Information (Per Serving):

- Carbs: 17 grams

- Fats: 19 grams

- Fiber: 4 grams

- Protein: 5 grams

Turkey and Vegetable Stir-Fry

Prep Time: 15 minutes
Cook Time: 15 minutes
Number of Servings: 4

Ingredients:

- 1 pound ground turkey

- 2 cups broccoli florets

- 1 red bell pepper, sliced

- 1 yellow bell pepper, sliced

- 1/2 cup snow peas, trimmed

- 1/2 cup sliced carrots

- 2 cloves garlic, minced

- 1 tablespoon fresh ginger, minced

- 2 tablespoons low-sodium soy sauce

- 1 tablespoon rice vinegar

- 1 teaspoon honey

- 1/2 teaspoon cornstarch

- 1/4 teaspoon crushed red pepper flakes (optional)

- 2 tablespoons sesame oil

- Cooked brown rice for serving

Instructions:

1. In a small bowl, whisk the low-sodium soy sauce, rice vinegar, honey, cornstarch, and crushed red pepper flakes if using. Set this sauce aside.

2. In a large wok or skillet, heat the sesame oil over medium-high heat.

3. Add the ground turkey to the heated wok and cook until it's browned and cooked through, breaking it into small pieces with a spatula. take out the turkey from the wok and set it aside.

4. In the same wok, add the minced garlic and ginger. Stir-fry for about 30 seconds until fragrant.

5. Add the broccoli, red bell pepper, yellow bell pepper, snow peas, and sliced carrots to the wok. Stir-fry for about 5-7 minutes or until the vegetables are tender-crisp.

6. Return the cooked turkey to the wok and pour the prepared sauce over the ingredients.

7. Stir-fry for an additional 2-3 minutes, ensuring the turkey and vegetables are well coated with the sauce and heated through.

8. Serve the turkey and vegetable stir-fry over cooked brown rice.

Nutritional Information (Per Serving):

- Carbs: 28 grams

- Fats: 13 grams

- Fiber: 5 grams

- Protein: 25 grams

Shrimp and Quinoa Pilaf

Prep Time: 15 minutes
Cook Time: 20 minutes
Number of Servings: 4

Ingredients:

- 1 cup quinoa, rinsed and drained
- 1 pound large shrimp, peeled and deveined
- 2 cups low-sodium chicken broth
- 1 red bell pepper, diced
- 1 yellow bell pepper, diced
- 1 small zucchini, diced
- 1 small yellow squash, diced
- 1/2 cup diced onion
- 2 cloves garlic, minced
- 1 teaspoon dried thyme
- 1/2 teaspoon ground cumin
- 1/2 teaspoon paprika
- 1/4 teaspoon black pepper
- 2 tablespoons olive oil
- Fresh parsley for garnish

Instructions:

1. In a large skillet, heat the olive oil over medium-high heat. Add the diced onion and cook for 2-3 minutes, or until it becomes translucent.

2. Add the minced garlic, dried thyme, ground cumin, paprika, and black pepper to the skillet. Stir and cook for an additional minute until fragrant.

3. Stir in the diced red and yellow bell peppers, zucchini, and yellow squash. Sauté for about 5 minutes or until the vegetables are tender-crisp.

4. Add the quinoa to the skillet and cook, stirring frequently, for about 2 minutes to lightly toast the quinoa.

5. Pour in the low-sodium chicken broth and bring the mixture to a boil. Reduce the heat to low, cover the skillet, and simmer for 15 minutes or until the quinoa is cooked and the liquid is absorbed.

6. While the quinoa is cooking, cook the shrimp. In a separate skillet, heat a bit of olive oil over medium-high heat. Add the shrimp and cook for 2-3 minutes per side until they turn pink and opaque.

7. Once the quinoa is cooked and the shrimp are done, add them in the skillet with the vegetable mixture. Gently stir to combine.

8. Serve the shrimp and quinoa pilaf garnished with fresh parsley.

Nutritional Information (Per Serving):

- Carbs: 45 grams

- Fats: 9 grams

- Fiber: 5 grams

- Protein: 30 grams

Spinach and Feta Stuffed Chicken Breast

Prep Time: 15 minutes
Cook Time: 25 minutes
Number of Servings: 4

Ingredients:

- 4 boneless, skinless chicken breasts

- 2 cups fresh spinach, chopped

- 1/2 cup crumbled feta cheese

- 1/4 cup diced sun-dried tomatoes

- 2 cloves garlic, minced

- 1/2 teaspoon dried oregano

- 1/2 teaspoon dried basil

- 1/4 teaspoon black pepper

- Olive oil for cooking

- Toothpicks or kitchen twine (to secure chicken)

Instructions:

1. Preheat your oven to 375°F (190°C).

2. In a mixing bowl, add the chopped fresh spinach, crumbled feta cheese, diced sun-dried tomatoes, minced garlic, dried oregano, dried basil, and black pepper. This mixture will be your stuffing.

3. Lay each chicken breast flat on a clean surface. Slice a pocket into the side of each chicken breast, being careful not to cut all the way through.

4. Stuff each chicken breast with the spinach and feta mixture, dividing it evenly among them. Secure the pockets closed with toothpicks or kitchen twine.

5. Heat a bit of olive oil in an oven-safe skillet over medium-high heat. Once hot, add the stuffed chicken breasts and cook for 3-4 minutes per side, or until they are browned.

6. Transfer the skillet to the preheated oven and bake for about 15-20 minutes, or until the chicken reaches an internal temperature of 165°F (74°C) and is no longer pink in the center.

7. Once cooked, take out the toothpicks or twine from the chicken breasts.

8. Serve the stuffed chicken breasts with any remaining spinach and feta mixture from the skillet.

Nutritional Information (Per Serving):

- Carbs: 5 grams

- Fats: 11 grams

- Fiber: 2 grams

- Protein: 37 grams

Lentil and Mushroom Meatballs

Prep Time: 20 minutes
Cook Time: 25 minutes
Number of Servings: 4

Ingredients:

- 1 cup dried green or brown lentils

- 2 cups water

- 1 cup cremini mushrooms, finely diced

- 1/2 cup rolled oats

- 1/4 cup grated Parmesan cheese

- 1/4 cup finely chopped onion

- 2 cloves garlic, minced

- 1 teaspoon dried oregano

- 1/2 teaspoon dried thyme

- 1/2 teaspoon dried basil

- 1/4 teaspoon black pepper

- 1/4 teaspoon salt

- 1 egg

- 2 tablespoons olive oil

- Marinara sauce for serving (optional)

Instructions:

1. In a medium saucepan, add the dried lentils and water. Bring to a boil, then reduce the heat to low, cover, and simmer for 20-25 minutes, or until the lentils are tender but not mushy. Drain any excess water and let the lentils cool.

2. In a large mixing bowl, add the cooked lentils, finely diced cremini mushrooms, rolled oats, grated Parmesan cheese, finely chopped onion, minced garlic, dried oregano, dried thyme, dried basil, black pepper, and salt.

3. Add the egg to the mixture and mix sufficiently to add all the ingredients.

4. Preheat your oven to 375°F (190°C).

5. Form the lentil and mushroom mixture into meatballs, approximately 1.5 inches in diameter, and place them on a baking sheet lined with parchment paper.

6. Brush the meatballs with olive oil to help them brown during baking.

7. Bake the meatballs in the preheated oven for about 20-25 minutes, or until they are firm and slightly browned.

8. Serve the lentil and mushroom meatballs with marinara sauce if desired.

Nutritional Information (Per Serving):

- Carbs: 27 grams

- Fats: 8 grams

- Fiber: 7 grams

- Protein: 13 grams

Teriyaki Tofu and Broccoli

Prep Time: 15 minutes
Cook Time: 20 minutes
Number of Servings: 4

Ingredients:

- 14 ounces extra-firm tofu, pressed and diced
- 2 cups broccoli florets
- 1/2 cup low-sodium soy sauce
- 1/4 cup water
- 2 tablespoons honey
- 2 tablespoons rice vinegar
- 2 cloves garlic, minced
- 1 teaspoon fresh ginger, minced
- 1 tablespoon cornstarch
- 1 tablespoon sesame oil
- 2 cups cooked brown rice
- Sesame seeds for garnish (optional)

Instructions:

1. In a small bowl, whisk the low-sodium soy sauce, water, honey, rice vinegar, minced garlic, minced ginger, and cornstarch. This mixture will be your teriyaki sauce.

2. Heat the sesame oil in a large skillet or wok over medium-high heat.

3. Add the diced extra-firm tofu to the hot skillet. Stir-fry for about 5-7 minutes or until the tofu is golden and slightly crispy. take out the tofu from the skillet and set it aside.

4. In the same skillet, add the broccoli florets and stir-fry for about 3-4 minutes, or until they become bright green and tender-crisp.

5. Return the cooked tofu to the skillet with the broccoli.

6. Pour the prepared teriyaki sauce over the tofu and broccoli. Stir-fry for an additional 2-3 minutes, or until the sauce thickens and coats the tofu and broccoli.

7. Serve the teriyaki tofu and broccoli over cooked brown rice and garnish with sesame seeds if desired.

Nutritional Information (Per Serving):

- Carbs: 44 grams

- Fats: 9 grams

- Fiber: 5 grams

- Protein: 15 grams

Baked Cod with Mediterranean Salsa

Prep Time: 15 minutes
Cook Time: 15 minutes
Number of Servings: 4

Ingredients:

- 4 cod fillets (about 1.5 pounds)

- 2 cups diced tomatoes

- 1/2 cup diced cucumber

- 1/4 cup chopped red onion

- 1/4 cup chopped Kalamata olives

- 2 tablespoons fresh basil, chopped

- 2 tablespoons fresh parsley, chopped

- 1 tablespoon olive oil

- 1 tablespoon balsamic vinegar

- 1 clove garlic, minced

- Salt and pepper to taste

- Lemon wedges for garnish (optional)

Instructions:

1. Preheat your oven to 400°F (200°C).

2. In a bowl, add the diced tomatoes, diced cucumber, chopped red onion, chopped Kalamata olives, fresh basil, and fresh parsley. This mixture will be your Mediterranean salsa.

3. In a separate small bowl, whisk the olive oil, balsamic vinegar, minced garlic, salt, and pepper to create the dressing.

4. Drizzle the dressing over the Mediterranean salsa and toss to combine. Set the salsa aside.

5. Place the cod fillets in a baking dish.

6. Spoon the Mediterranean salsa over the cod fillets, ensuring they are well covered.

7. Bake in the preheated oven for about 15 minutes or until the cod is opaque and flakes easily with a fork.

8. Serve the baked cod with Mediterranean salsa and garnish with lemon wedges if desired.

Nutritional Information (Per Serving):

- Carbs: 8 grams

- Fats: 6 grams

- Fiber: 2 grams

- Protein: 34 grams

Ratatouille with Chickpeas

Prep Time: 15 minutes
Cook Time: 30 minutes
Number of Servings: 4

Ingredients:

- 2 tablespoons olive oil

- 1 onion, diced

- 2 cloves garlic, minced

- 1 eggplant, diced

- 2 zucchinis, diced

- 1 red bell pepper, diced

- 1 yellow bell pepper, diced

- 1 can (15 ounces) chickpeas, drained and rinsed

- 1 can (15 ounces) diced tomatoes

- 2 teaspoons dried thyme

- 1 teaspoon dried rosemary

- Salt and pepper to taste

- Fresh basil for garnish

Instructions:

1. In a large skillet, heat the olive oil over medium heat.

2. Add the diced onion and cook for 2-3 minutes until it becomes translucent.

3. Stir in the minced garlic and cook for an additional 30 seconds until fragrant.

4. Add the diced eggplant, zucchinis, red bell pepper, and yellow bell pepper to the skillet. Sauté for about 5-7 minutes, or until the vegetables start to soften.

5. Mix in the drained and rinsed chickpeas, diced tomatoes, dried thyme, dried rosemary, salt, and pepper. Stir sufficiently to add all the ingredients.

6. Cover the skillet and simmer for approximately 15-20 minutes, or until the vegetables are tender and the flavors have melded.

7. Taste and adjust the seasoning with additional salt and pepper if needed.

8. Serve the ratatouille with chickpeas garnished with fresh basil.

Nutritional Information (Per Serving):

- Carbs: 40 grams

- Fats: 6 grams

- Fiber: 11 grams

- Protein: 11 grams

Lemon Dill Grilled Trout

Prep Time: 15 minutes
Cook Time: 10 minutes
Number of Servings: 4

Ingredients:

- 4 trout fillets (about 1.5 pounds)

- 2 lemons, zested and juiced

- 2 tablespoons olive oil

- 2 tablespoons fresh dill, chopped

- 1 teaspoon dried oregano

- 1/2 teaspoon garlic powder

- Salt and pepper to taste

- Lemon wedges for serving

Instructions:

1. Preheat your grill to medium-high heat.

2. In a small bowl, add the lemon zest, lemon juice, olive oil, chopped fresh dill, dried oregano, garlic powder, salt, and pepper. This mixture will be your marinade.

3. Place the trout fillets on a large plate or in a shallow dish. Pour the marinade over the fillets, ensuring they are well coated. Let them marinate for at least 15 minutes, turning occasionally.

4. Grease the grill grates to prevent sticking.

5. Place the marinated trout fillets on the preheated grill. Cook for about 4-5 minutes per side or until the fish flakes easily with a fork and is no longer translucent in the center.

6. While grilling, you can baste the trout fillets with any remaining marinade for extra flavor.

7. Once cooked, take out the trout fillets from the grill and let them rest for a few minutes.

8. Serve the lemon dill grilled trout with lemon wedges for an extra burst of fresh citrus flavor.

Nutritional Information (Per Serving):

- Carbs: 3 grams

- Fats: 9 grams

- Fiber: 1 gram

- Protein: 24 grams

Pesto Zucchini Noodles with Cherry Tomatoes

Prep Time: 15 minutes
Cook Time: 5 minutes
Number of Servings: 4

Ingredients:

- 4 medium-sized zucchinis
- 1 pint cherry tomatoes, halved
- 1/2 cup pesto sauce
- 1/4 cup grated Parmesan cheese
- 2 tablespoons pine nuts
- 2 tablespoons olive oil
- Salt and pepper to taste
- Fresh basil leaves for garnish (optional)

Instructions:

1. Using a spiralizer or a julienne peeler, create zucchini noodles from the four medium-sized zucchinis. Set the zucchini noodles aside.

2. In a large skillet, heat the olive oil over medium heat.

3. Add the cherry tomatoes to the skillet and sauté for about 2-3 minutes, or until they begin to soften and release some juices.

4. Add the zucchini noodles to the skillet and toss them with the cherry tomatoes. Sauté for an additional 2-3 minutes, or until the zucchini noodles are just tender but still slightly crisp.

5. Stir in the pesto sauce and toss to coat the zucchini noodles and cherry tomatoes evenly.

6. Take out the skillet from the heat.

7. Serve the pesto zucchini noodles with cherry tomatoes topped with grated Parmesan cheese and pine nuts.

8. Garnish with fresh basil leaves if desired.

Nutritional Information (Per Serving):

- Carbs: 14 grams

- Fats: 25 grams

- Fiber: 3 grams

- Protein: 8 grams

Eggplant Parmesan

Prep Time: 30 minutes
Cook Time: 40 minutes
Number of Servings: 4

Ingredients:

- 2 large eggplants, sliced into 1/2-inch rounds

- 2 cups marinara sauce (low-sodium)

- 1 1/2 cups part-skim mozzarella cheese, shredded

- 1/2 cup grated Parmesan cheese

- 1 cup whole-wheat bread crumbs

- 1/2 cup all-purpose flour

- 2 large eggs

- 2 teaspoons dried oregano

- 2 teaspoons dried basil

- 1/2 teaspoon garlic powder

- Olive oil for frying

- Salt and pepper to taste

- Fresh basil leaves for garnish (optional)

Instructions:

1. Start by preparing an assembly line for coating the eggplant slices. In one shallow dish, place the all-purpose flour. In an extra, whisk the eggs. In a third dish, add the whole-wheat bread crumbs, dried oregano, dried basil, garlic powder, salt, and pepper.

2. Take each eggplant slice and coat it first in the flour, then dip it in the beaten eggs, and finally, coat it in the bread crumb mixture. Set the coated slices aside on a baking sheet.

3. In a large skillet, heat enough olive oil to cover the bottom of the pan over medium-high heat. Once the oil is hot, add the breaded eggplant slices and fry until golden brown on both sides. Place the fried slices on a paper towel-lined plate to remove excess oil.

4. Preheat your oven to 375°F (190°C).

5. In a baking dish, spread a thin layer of marinara sauce. Place a layer of fried eggplant slices on top of the sauce.

6. Sprinkle mozzarella and Parmesan cheese over the eggplant layer, and then add more marinara sauce on top.

7. Repeat the layering process with the remaining eggplant slices, cheese, and sauce.

8. Bake in the preheated oven for about 20-25 minutes, or until the cheese is bubbly and golden brown.

9. Garnish with fresh basil leaves if desired.

Nutritional Information (Per Serving):

- Carbs: 40 grams

- Fats: 17 grams

- Fiber: 10 grams

- Protein: 20 grams

Quinoa and Black Bean Stuffed Bell Peppers

Prep Time: 20 minutes
Cook Time: 40 minutes
Number of Servings: 4

Ingredients:

- 4 large bell peppers (any color)

- 1 cup quinoa, rinsed

- 2 cups low-sodium vegetable broth

- 1 can (15 ounces) black beans, drained and rinsed

- 1 cup corn kernels (fresh, frozen, or canned)

- 1 cup diced tomatoes

- 1/2 cup diced red onion

- 2 cloves garlic, minced

- 2 teaspoons chili powder

- 1 teaspoon ground cumin

- 1/2 teaspoon paprika

- Salt and pepper to taste

- 1 cup shredded low-fat cheddar cheese

- Chopped fresh cilantro for garnish (optional)

Instructions:

1. Preheat your oven to 375°F (190°C).

2. Slice the tops off the bell peppers and take out the seeds and membranes. Set them aside.

3. In a large saucepan, add the quinoa and low-sodium vegetable broth. Bring to a boil, then reduce the heat to low, cover, and

simmer for about 15 minutes, or until the quinoa is cooked and the liquid is absorbed.

4. In a large mixing bowl, add the cooked quinoa, black beans, corn kernels, diced tomatoes, diced red onion, minced garlic, chili powder, ground cumin, paprika, salt, and pepper.

5. Stuff each bell pepper with the quinoa and black bean mixture.

6. Place the stuffed bell peppers in a baking dish and cover it with aluminum foil.

7. Bake in the preheated oven for about 25-30 minutes, or until the bell peppers are tender.

8.   Take out the foil, sprinkle shredded low-fat cheddar cheese over the tops of the bell peppers, and return them to the oven. Bake for an additional 5-10 minutes, or until the cheese is melted and bubbly.

9. Garnish with chopped fresh cilantro if desired.

Nutritional Information (Per Serving):

- Carbs: 54 grams

- Fats: 5 grams

- Fiber: 12 grams

- Protein: 15 grams

Grilled Lemon Dill Swordfish

Prep Time: 15 minutes
Cook Time: 10 minutes
Number of Servings: 4

Ingredients:

- 4 swordfish steaks (about 6 ounces each)

- Zest and juice of 1 lemon

- 2 tablespoons olive oil

- 2 tablespoons fresh dill, chopped

- 2 cloves garlic, minced

- Salt and black pepper to taste

- Lemon wedges for serving (optional)

Instructions:

1. Preheat your grill to medium-high heat.

2. In a small bowl, add the lemon zest, lemon juice, olive oil, chopped fresh dill, minced garlic, salt, and black pepper. This mixture will be your marinade.

3. Place the swordfish steaks in a shallow dish and pour the marinade over them. Make sure the steaks are well coated. Let them marinate for about 10-15 minutes.

4. Grease the grill grates to prevent sticking.

5. Take out the swordfish steaks from the marinade and grill them on the preheated grill. Grill for about 4-5 minutes per side, or until the fish is opaque and flakes easily with a fork.

6. While grilling, you can brush the swordfish steaks with any remaining marinade for extra flavor.

7. Serve the grilled lemon dill swordfish with lemon wedges for an additional burst of fresh citrus flavor if desired.

Nutritional Information (Per Serving):

- Carbs: 1 gram

- Fats: 11 grams

- Fiber: 0 grams

- Protein: 35 grams

Chickpea and Vegetable Curry

Prep Time: 15 minutes
Cook Time: 25 minutes
Number of Servings: 4

Ingredients:

- 1 cup dried chickpeas, soaked and cooked (or 2 cans, 15 ounces each, of canned chickpeas, drained and rinsed)

- 1 cup diced eggplant

- 1 cup diced zucchini

- 1 cup diced bell peppers (any color)

- 1 cup diced onion

- 2 cloves garlic, minced

- 1 can (14 ounces) diced tomatoes

- 1 can (14 ounces) light coconut milk

- 2 tablespoons olive oil

- 2 tablespoons curry powder

- 1 teaspoon ground cumin

- 1/2 teaspoon ground turmeric

- Salt and black pepper to taste

- Fresh cilantro for garnish (optional)

Instructions:

1. If using dried chickpeas, soak them overnight or for at least 8 hours. Cook the soaked chickpeas in a large pot of water until they are tender, which will take about 1-1.5 hours. If using canned chickpeas, make sure to drain and rinse them.

2. In a large skillet, heat the olive oil over medium heat.

3. Add the diced onion and cook for about 2-3 minutes until it becomes translucent.

4. Stir in the minced garlic, diced eggplant, diced zucchini, and diced bell peppers. Sauté for about 5-7 minutes, or until the vegetables start to soften.

5. Add the curry powder, ground cumin, ground turmeric, salt, and black pepper to the skillet. Stir sufficiently to coat the vegetables with the spices.

6. Pour in the diced tomatoes (with their juice) and light coconut milk. Mix everything together.

7. Let the mixture simmer for about 10-15 minutes, or until the vegetables are tender and the flavors have melded.

8. Add the cooked or canned chickpeas to the skillet and heat them through for an additional 5 minutes.

9. Serve the chickpea and vegetable curry hot, garnished with fresh cilantro if desired.

Nutritional Information (Per Serving):

- Carbs: 35 grams

- Fats: 9 grams

- Fiber: 10 grams

- Protein: 11 grams

Turkey and Sweet Potato Shepherd's Pie

Prep Time: 25 minutes
Cook Time: 25 minutes
Number of Servings: 6

Ingredients:

- 1 pound lean ground turkey

- 2 cups sweet potatoes, peeled and diced
- 1 cup carrots, diced
- 1 cup peas
- 1 cup corn
- 1 onion, diced
- 2 cloves garlic, minced
- 1 cup low-sodium chicken broth
- 2 tablespoons tomato paste
- 1 tablespoon olive oil
- 1 teaspoon dried thyme
- 1/2 teaspoon dried rosemary
- Salt and black pepper to taste

Instructions:

1. Preheat your oven to 375°F (190°C).

2. Place the sweet potato pieces in a large pot of water. Bring the water to a boil and cook the sweet potatoes for about 15 minutes, or until they are tender.

3. While the sweet potatoes are cooking, heat the olive oil in a large skillet over medium heat.

4. Add the diced onion and cook for about 2-3 minutes until it becomes translucent.

5. Stir in the minced garlic and cook for an additional 30 seconds until fragrant.

6. Add the ground turkey to the skillet and cook until it's no longer pink, breaking it up with a spoon as it cooks.

7. Add the diced carrots, peas, corn, dried thyme, dried rosemary, salt, and black pepper to the skillet. Cook for about 5-7 minutes until the vegetables start to soften.

8. Mix in the tomato paste and low-sodium chicken broth. Stir sufficiently and simmer for an additional 5 minutes, or until the mixture thickens slightly.

9. Drain and mash the cooked sweet potatoes.

10. Transfer the turkey and vegetable mixture to a baking dish and spread the mashed sweet potatoes on top.

11. Place the baking dish in the preheated oven and bake for about 20-25 minutes, or until the top is golden and the filling is bubbling.

12. Serve the turkey and sweet potato shepherd's pie hot.

Nutritional Information (Per Serving):

- Carbs: 27 grams

- Fats: 6 grams

- Fiber: 5 grams

- Protein: 19 grams

Quinoa-Stuffed Bell Peppers with Turkey

Prep Time: 20 minutes
Cook Time: 45 minutes
Number of Servings: 4

Ingredients:

- 4 large bell peppers (any color)

- 1 cup quinoa, rinsed

- 1 pound lean ground turkey

- 1 can (14 ounces) diced tomatoes

- 1/2 cup low-sodium chicken broth

- 1/2 cup diced onion

- 1/2 cup diced zucchini

- 1/2 cup diced red bell pepper

- 2 cloves garlic, minced

- 1 teaspoon dried oregano

- 1 teaspoon dried basil

- 1/2 teaspoon chili powder

- 1/2 teaspoon black pepper

- Salt to taste

- 1 cup low-fat mozzarella cheese, shredded

- Chopped fresh parsley for garnish (optional)

Instructions:

1. Preheat your oven to 375°F (190°C).

2. Slice the tops off the bell peppers and take out the seeds and membranes. Set them aside.

3. In a large saucepan, add the quinoa and two cups of water. Bring to a boil, then reduce the heat to low, cover, and simmer for about 15 minutes, or until the quinoa is cooked and the water is absorbed.

4. In a large skillet, cook the ground turkey over medium heat until it's no longer pink, breaking it up with a spoon as it cooks. Drain any excess fat.

5. Stir in the diced onion, diced zucchini, diced red bell pepper, and minced garlic. Sauté for about 5-7 minutes, or until the vegetables start to soften.

6. Add the cooked quinoa, diced tomatoes, low-sodium chicken broth, dried oregano, dried basil, chili powder, black pepper, and salt to

the skillet. Mix everything together and let it simmer for about 5 minutes.

7. Fill each bell pepper with the quinoa and turkey mixture.

8. Place the stuffed bell peppers in a baking dish and cover it with aluminum foil.

9. Bake in the preheated oven for about 30 minutes, or until the bell peppers are tender.

10. Take out the foil, sprinkle low-fat mozzarella cheese over the tops of the bell peppers, and return them to the oven. Bake for an additional 10-15 minutes, or until the cheese is melted and bubbly.

11.Garnish with chopped fresh parsley if desired.

Nutritional Information (Per Serving):

- Carbs: 44 grams

- Fats: 11 grams

- Fiber: 6 grams

- Protein: 30 grams

Balsamic Glazed Salmon

Prep Time: 10 minutes
Cook Time: 15 minutes
Number of Servings: 4

Ingredients:

- 4 salmon fillets (about 6 ounces each)

- 1/4 cup balsamic vinegar

- 2 tablespoons honey

- 2 tablespoons low-sodium soy sauce

- 2 cloves garlic, minced

- 1 tablespoon olive oil

- 1/2 teaspoon dried rosemary

- Salt and black pepper to taste

- Fresh rosemary sprigs for garnish (optional)

Instructions:

1. In a small bowl, whisk the balsamic vinegar, honey, low-sodium soy sauce, minced garlic, dried rosemary, salt, and black pepper. This mixture will be your glaze.

2. Heat the olive oil in a large skillet over medium-high heat.

3. Season the salmon fillets with a little salt and black pepper.

4. Place the salmon fillets in the skillet, skin side down. Cook for about 4-5 minutes, or until the skin is crispy and the salmon easily releases from the pan.

5. Flip the salmon fillets and cook for an additional 2-3 minutes.

6. Pour the balsamic glaze over the salmon in the skillet.

7. Continue cooking the salmon for an extra 2-3 minutes, or until it's cooked to your desired level of doneness and the glaze has thickened.

8. Spoon the glaze from the skillet over the salmon as it cooks.

9. Once the salmon is cooked to your liking and the glaze is sticky, take it out of the heat.

10. Garnish with fresh rosemary sprigs if desired.

Nutritional Information (Per Serving):

- Carbs: 14 grams

- Fats: 14 grams

- Fiber: 0 grams

- Protein: 37 grams

Tofu and Vegetable Kebabs with Peanut Sauce

Prep Time: 30 minutes
Cook Time: 15 minutes
Number of Servings: 4

Ingredients:

For the Kebabs:

- 14 ounces extra-firm tofu, cubed

- 1 red bell pepper, diced

- 1 yellow bell pepper, diced

- 1 red onion, diced

- 1 zucchini, sliced into rounds

- 8 wooden skewers (soaked in water for at least 30 minutes)

For the Marinade:

- 1/4 cup low-sodium soy sauce

- 2 tablespoons olive oil

- 2 cloves garlic, minced

- 1 teaspoon ground ginger

- 1 teaspoon sesame oil

- 1/2 teaspoon black pepper

For the Peanut Sauce:

- 1/4 cup natural peanut butter

- 2 tablespoons low-sodium soy sauce

- 2 tablespoons water

- 1 tablespoon lime juice

- 1 tablespoon honey
- 1 teaspoon Sriracha sauce (adjust to taste)

Instructions:

1. In a bowl, whisk the ingredients for the marinade: low-sodium soy sauce, olive oil, minced garlic, ground ginger, sesame oil, and black pepper.

2. Thread the tofu cubes, diced red and yellow bell peppers, diced red onion, and zucchini rounds onto the soaked wooden skewers, alternating the ingredients as desired.

3. Place the assembled kebabs in a shallow dish and brush them with the marinade. Allow them to marinate for at least 15-20 minutes.

4. While the kebabs are marinating, preheat your grill to medium-high heat.

5. In a small saucepan, add the ingredients for the peanut sauce: natural peanut butter, low-sodium soy sauce, water, lime juice, honey, and Sriracha sauce. Heat over low heat, stirring until the sauce is smooth and well combined. Set aside.

6. Grease the grill grates to prevent sticking.

7. Grill the tofu and vegetable kebabs for about 10-15 minutes, turning occasionally, until the vegetables are tender and the tofu is lightly charred.

8. Serve the kebabs with the peanut sauce for dipping.

Nutritional Information (Per Serving):

- Carbs: 19 grams
- Fats: 16 grams
- Fiber: 3 grams
- Protein: 13 grams

Mediterranean Baked Cod

Prep Time: 15 minutes
Cook Time: 20 minutes
Number of Servings: 4

Ingredients:

- 4 cod fillets (about 6 ounces each)
- 1 cup cherry tomatoes
- 1/2 cup Kalamata olives, pitted and sliced
- 1/2 cup red onion, thinly sliced
- 4 cloves garlic, minced
- 2 tablespoons extra-virgin olive oil
- 1 tablespoon balsamic vinegar
- 1 teaspoon dried oregano
- 1/2 teaspoon dried basil
- 1/2 teaspoon dried thyme
- Salt and black pepper to taste
- Fresh parsley for garnish (optional)
- Lemon wedges for serving (optional)

Instructions:

1. Preheat your oven to 375°F (190°C).

2. In a large mixing bowl, add the cherry tomatoes, Kalamata olives, thinly sliced red onion, minced garlic, extra-virgin olive oil, balsamic vinegar, dried oregano, dried basil, dried thyme, salt, and black pepper. This mixture will be your Mediterranean topping.

3. Place the cod fillets in a baking dish.

4. Spoon the Mediterranean topping over the cod fillets, ensuring to distribute it evenly.

5. Cover the baking dish with aluminum foil.

6. Bake in the preheated oven for about 15-20 minutes, or until the cod is opaque and flakes easily with a fork.

7.   Take out the foil and broil for an additional 2-3 minutes, or until the topping is slightly charred.

8. Garnish with fresh parsley and serve with lemon wedges if desired.

Nutritional Information (Per Serving):

- Carbs: 7 grams

- Fats: 11 grams

- Fiber: 2 grams

- Protein: 28 grams

Spaghetti Squash with Roasted Cherry Tomatoes

Prep Time: 10 minutes
Cook Time: 45 minutes
Number of Servings: 4

Ingredients:

- 1 spaghetti squash

- 2 cups cherry tomatoes

- 2 tablespoons olive oil

- 4 cloves garlic, minced

- 1/4 cup fresh basil, chopped

- 1/4 cup fresh parsley, chopped

- Salt and black pepper to taste

- Grated Parmesan cheese for garnish (optional)

Instructions:

1. Preheat your oven to 375°F (190°C).

2. Carefully cut the spaghetti squash in half lengthwise and take out the seeds and pulp.

3. Drizzle the cut sides of the spaghetti squash with one tablespoon of olive oil and season with a bit of salt and black pepper.

4. Place the spaghetti squash halves, cut side down, on a baking sheet and roast in the preheated oven for about 35-40 minutes, or until the flesh is tender and easily shreds with a fork.

5. While the spaghetti squash is roasting, toss the cherry tomatoes with the remaining one tablespoon of olive oil, minced garlic, and some salt and black pepper.

6. Place the seasoned cherry tomatoes on a separate baking sheet and roast in the oven alongside the spaghetti squash for about 20-25 minutes, or until they are soft and slightly blistered.

7. Once the spaghetti squash is done, use a fork to shred the flesh into "spaghetti" strands.

8. Mix the roasted cherry tomatoes, fresh basil, and fresh parsley into the shredded spaghetti squash.

9. Taste and adjust the seasoning with more salt and black pepper if needed.

10. Serve the spaghetti squash with roasted cherry tomatoes as a side dish, and garnish with grated Parmesan cheese if desired.

Nutritional Information (Per Serving):

- Carbs: 15 grams

- Fats: 7 grams

- Fiber: 3 grams

- Protein: 2 grams

Chapter 7: Side Dishes

Roasted Asparagus with Lemon Zest

Prep Time: 10 minutes
Cook Time: 15 minutes
Number of Servings: 4

Ingredients:

- 1 pound fresh asparagus spears, trimmed
- 1 lemon, zest and juice
- 2 cloves garlic, minced
- 2 tablespoons olive oil
- 1/4 teaspoon salt
- 1/4 teaspoon black pepper

Instructions:

1. Preheat your oven to 425°F (220°C).

2. In a small bowl, add the olive oil, minced garlic, lemon zest, lemon juice, salt, and black pepper.

3. Place the trimmed asparagus spears on a baking sheet and drizzle the lemon and garlic mixture over them. Toss the asparagus to ensure they are evenly coated.

4. Spread the asparagus in a single layer on the baking sheet.

5. Roast in the preheated oven for 12-15 minutes or until the asparagus is tender and slightly browned, giving them a gentle stir halfway through.

6. Once roasted to your desired tenderness, take out the asparagus from the oven.

7. Serve hot and garnish with a little extra lemon zest, if desired.

Nutritional Information (per serving):

- Carbs: 7 grams

- Fats: 7 grams

- Fiber: 3 grams

- Protein: 3 grams

Garlic and Herb Quinoa

Prep Time: 10 minutes
Cook Time: 20 minutes
Number of Servings: 4

Ingredients:

- 1 cup quinoa

- 2 cups low-sodium vegetable broth

- 3 cloves garlic, minced

- 1 tablespoon olive oil

- 1/2 teaspoon dried thyme

- 1/2 teaspoon dried rosemary

- 1/2 teaspoon dried basil

- 1/4 teaspoon salt

- 1/4 teaspoon black pepper

Instructions:

1. Rinse the quinoa thoroughly under cold water to take out any bitterness. Drain well.

2. In a medium saucepan, heat the olive oil over medium heat. Add the minced garlic and sauté for about 1 minute until fragrant.

3. Add the rinsed quinoa to the saucepan with the garlic and sauté for an extra 2 minutes, stirring occasionally.

4. Pour in the low-sodium vegetable broth and add the dried thyme, dried rosemary, dried basil, salt, and black pepper. Stir to combine.

5. Bring the mixture to a boil. Once boiling, reduce the heat to low, cover the saucepan, and simmer for 15-20 minutes or until the quinoa is cooked and the liquid is absorbed.

6. Take out the saucepan from heat and let it sit, covered, for 5 minutes to allow the quinoa to fluff up.

7. Fluff the quinoa with a fork and serve hot.

Nutritional Information (per serving):

- Carbs: 37 grams

- Fats: 5 grams

- Fiber: 3 grams

- Protein: 7 grams

Green Beans Almondine

Prep Time: 10 minutes
Cook Time: 15 minutes
Number of Servings: 4

Ingredients:

- 1 pound fresh green beans, ends trimmed

- 1/4 cup sliced almonds

- 1 tablespoon olive oil

- 2 cloves garlic, minced

- 1/2 tablespoon lemon juice

- 1/4 teaspoon salt

- 1/4 teaspoon black pepper

Instructions:

1. Bring a large pot of water to a boil. Add the trimmed green beans and blanch them for about 2-3 minutes or until they are tender-crisp. Drain and immediately transfer to a bowl of ice water to stop the cooking process. Drain again and set aside.

2. In a large skillet, heat the olive oil over medium heat. Add the sliced almonds and toast them for 2-3 minutes or until they turn golden brown. Stir them frequently to prevent burning. take out the toasted almonds from the skillet and set them aside.

3. In the same skillet, add the minced garlic and sauté for about 1 minute until fragrant.

4. Add the blanched green beans to the skillet with the garlic. Toss them to add and heat for an additional 2 minutes.

5. Drizzle the lemon juice over the green beans and season with salt and black pepper. Toss to coat the beans evenly.

6. Transfer the green beans almondine to a serving dish, and sprinkle the toasted almonds over the top.

7. Serve hot.

Nutritional Information (per serving):

- Carbs: 9 grams

- Fats: 7 grams

- Fiber: 4 grams

- Protein: 3 grams

Sautéed Kale with Garlic

Prep Time: 10 minutes
Cook Time: 10 minutes
Number of Servings: 4

Ingredients:

- 1 bunch fresh kale, stems Take outd and leaves chopped
- 2 cloves garlic, minced
- 1 tablespoon olive oil
- 1/4 teaspoon red pepper flakes (optional)
- 1/4 teaspoon salt
- 1/4 teaspoon black pepper
- 1 tablespoon lemon juice

Instructions:

1. Start by preparing the kale. Wash the kale leaves thoroughly, take out the tough stems, and chop the leaves into bite-sized pieces.

2. In a large skillet, heat the olive oil over medium heat.

3. Add the minced garlic and red pepper flakes (if using) to the skillet. Sauté for about 1 minute or until the garlic becomes fragrant.

4. Add the chopped kale to the skillet. It may seem like a lot, but it will wilt as it cooks.

5. Sauté the kale, stirring frequently, for about 5-7 minutes or until it is tender and has reduced in volume.

6. Season the sautéed kale with salt and black pepper. Stir to combine.

7. Drizzle the lemon juice over the kale and toss it to distribute the flavors evenly.

8. Transfer the sautéed kale to a serving dish.

9. Serve hot.

Nutritional Information (per serving):

- Carbs: 8 grams

- Fats: 3 grams

- Fiber: 2 grams

- Protein: 2 grams

Cilantro Lime Brown Rice

Prep Time: 10 minutes
Cook Time: 45 minutes
Number of Servings: 4

Ingredients:

- 1 cup brown rice

- 2 cups low-sodium vegetable broth

- 2 cloves garlic, minced

- 2 tablespoons fresh cilantro, finely chopped

- 1 tablespoon olive oil

- 1 tablespoon lime juice

- 1/4 teaspoon salt

- 1/4 teaspoon black pepper

- 1 lime, cut into wedges for garnish

Instructions:

1. Rinse the brown rice thoroughly under cold water to remove excess starch. Drain well.

2. In a medium saucepan, heat the olive oil over medium heat. Add the minced garlic and sauté for about 1 minute until fragrant.

3. Add the rinsed brown rice to the saucepan with the garlic and sauté for an extra 2 minutes, stirring occasionally.

4. Pour in the low-sodium vegetable broth and bring it to a boil.

5. Reduce the heat to low, cover the saucepan, and simmer for 45 minutes or until the rice is tender and the liquid is absorbed.

6. Once the rice is cooked, fluff it with a fork.

7. Add the finely chopped cilantro, lime juice, salt, and black pepper. Stir to combine, allowing the flavors to meld.

8. Serve the Cilantro Lime Brown Rice with lime wedges for garnish.

Nutritional Information (per serving):

- Carbs: 41 grams

- Fats: 3 grams

- Fiber: 3 grams

- Protein: 4 grams

Balsamic Roasted Brussels Sprouts

Prep Time: 10 minutes
Cook Time: 25 minutes
Number of Servings: 4

Ingredients:

- 1 pound fresh Brussels sprouts, trimmed and halved

- 2 tablespoons olive oil

- 2 tablespoons balsamic vinegar

- 2 cloves garlic, minced

- 1/4 teaspoon salt

- 1/4 teaspoon black pepper

Instructions:

1. Preheat your oven to 425°F (220°C).

2. In a mixing bowl, add the olive oil, balsamic vinegar, minced garlic, salt, and black pepper.

3. Place the trimmed and halved Brussels sprouts on a baking sheet.

4. Drizzle the balsamic mixture over the Brussels sprouts and toss them to ensure they are evenly coated.

5. Spread the Brussels sprouts out in a single layer on the baking sheet.

6. Roast in the preheated oven for 20-25 minutes or until the Brussels sprouts are tender and slightly caramelized, stirring once or twice during roasting.

7. Once roasted to your desired tenderness, take out the Brussels sprouts from the oven.

8. Serve hot.

Nutritional Information (per serving):

- Carbs: 12 grams

- Fats: 7 grams

- Fiber: 4 grams

- Protein: 3 grams

Grilled Corn on the Cob with Chili-Lime Butter

Prep Time: 10 minutes
Cook Time: 15 minutes
Number of Servings: 4

Ingredients:

- 4 ears of fresh corn, husked

- 2 tablespoons unsalted butter, softened

- 1 teaspoon chili powder

- 1/2 teaspoon lime zest

- 1 tablespoon fresh lime juice

- 1/4 teaspoon salt

- 1/4 teaspoon black pepper

Instructions:

1. Preheat your grill to medium-high heat.

2. In a small bowl, prepare the chili-lime butter. Add the softened unsalted butter, chili powder, lime zest, lime juice, salt, and black pepper. Mix until all the ingredients are well incorporated.

3. Place each ear of corn on a piece of aluminum foil. Spread the chili-lime butter mixture evenly over each ear of corn.

4. Wrap each ear of corn securely in the aluminum foil.

5. Grill the corn on the preheated grill for about 12-15 minutes, turning occasionally, until the corn is tender and has grill marks.

6. Carefully unwrap the grilled corn and serve hot.

Nutritional Information (per serving):

- Carbs: 32 grams

- Fats: 6 grams

- Fiber: 4 grams

- Protein: 4 grams

Lemon Garlic Roasted Potatoes

Prep Time: 10 minutes
Cook Time: 40 minutes
Number of Servings: 4

Ingredients:

- 1.5 pounds (about 680 grams) small red potatoes, washed and quartered

- 2 tablespoons olive oil

- 4 cloves garlic, minced

- 1 tablespoon fresh lemon juice

- 1 teaspoon lemon zest

- 1/4 teaspoon salt

- 1/4 teaspoon black pepper

- 2 tablespoons fresh parsley, chopped for garnish

Instructions:

1. Preheat your oven to 425°F (220°C).

2. In a large bowl, add the quartered red potatoes, olive oil, minced garlic, lemon juice, lemon zest, salt, and black pepper. Toss to ensure the potatoes are evenly coated with the mixture.

3. Spread the seasoned potatoes in a single layer on a baking sheet.

4. Roast in the preheated oven for 35-40 minutes or until the potatoes are golden brown and tender. Be sure to give them a stir or shake the pan a couple of times during roasting to ensure even cooking.

5. Once the potatoes are roasted to your desired tenderness, take them out of the oven.

6. Garnish with fresh chopped parsley before serving.

Nutritional Information (per serving):

- Carbs: 35 grams

- Fats: 7 grams

- Fiber: 3 grams

- Protein: 4 grams

Sesame Ginger Broccoli

Prep Time: 10 minutes
Cook Time: 10 minutes
Number of Servings: 4

Ingredients:

- 1 pound (about 450 grams) fresh broccoli florets

- 2 tablespoons low-sodium soy sauce

- 1 tablespoon sesame oil

- 2 teaspoons fresh ginger, minced

- 2 cloves garlic, minced

- 1/2 teaspoon honey

- 1/4 teaspoon sesame seeds (for garnish)

- 1/4 teaspoon red pepper flakes (optional, adjust to taste)

Instructions:

1. Steam or blanch the broccoli florets for about 3-4 minutes, just until they are tender-crisp. Drain and set aside.

2. In a small bowl, prepare the sauce by combining the low-sodium soy sauce, sesame oil, minced ginger, minced garlic, honey, and red pepper flakes (if using).

3. Heat a large skillet or wok over medium-high heat. Add the steamed broccoli to the skillet.

4. Pour the sesame ginger sauce over the broccoli in the skillet.

5. Stir-fry the broccoli for about 3-5 minutes, ensuring it is evenly coated with the sauce and heated through.

6. Once the broccoli is tender and has absorbed the flavors of the sauce, take it out of the heat.

7. Serve the Sesame Ginger Broccoli, garnished with sesame seeds.

Nutritional Information (per serving):

- Carbs: 8 grams

- Fats: 4 grams

- Fiber: 3 grams

- Protein: 3 grams

Cucumber and Red Onion Salad

Prep Time: 15 minutes
Cook Time: 0 minutes
Number of Servings: 4

Ingredients:

- 2 large cucumbers, thinly sliced

- 1/2 red onion, thinly sliced

- 2 tablespoons fresh dill, chopped

- 2 tablespoons olive oil

- 2 tablespoons red wine vinegar

- 1/4 teaspoon salt

- 1/4 teaspoon black pepper

Instructions:

1. In a large bowl, add the thinly sliced cucumbers and red onion.

2. In a small bowl, whisk the olive oil, red wine vinegar, salt, and black pepper to create the dressing.

3. Drizzle the dressing over the cucumber and red onion slices.

4. Add the fresh chopped dill to the bowl.

5. Gently toss all the ingredients to ensure the cucumber and red onion are evenly coated with the dressing.

6. Refrigerate the salad for about 15-20 minutes to let the flavors meld.

7. Before serving, toss the salad once more to redistribute the dressing.

8. Serve the Cucumber and Red Onion Salad chilled.

Nutritional Information (per serving):

- Carbs: 6 grams

- Fats: 7 grams

- Fiber: 1 gram

- Protein: 1 gram

Roasted Beet and Arugula Salad

Prep Time: 15 minutes
Cook Time: 45 minutes (for roasting beets)
Number of Servings: 4

Ingredients:

- 4 medium beets, trimmed and peeled

- 4 cups fresh arugula

- 1/4 cup crumbled feta cheese

- 1/4 cup walnuts, chopped

- 2 tablespoons olive oil

- 2 tablespoons balsamic vinegar

- 1/4 teaspoon salt

- 1/4 teaspoon black pepper

Instructions:

1. Preheat your oven to 400°F (200°C).

2. Place the trimmed and peeled beets on a baking sheet. Drizzle them with a little olive oil and wrap them in aluminum foil. Roast the beets in the preheated oven for about 45 minutes or until they are tender when pierced with a fork.

3. Allow the roasted beets to cool, then slice them into thin rounds or wedges.

4. In a large salad bowl, add the fresh arugula, roasted beet slices, and crumbled feta cheese.

5. In a small bowl, whisk the remaining olive oil, balsamic vinegar, salt, and black pepper to create the dressing.

6. Drizzle the dressing over the salad and toss gently to ensure the ingredients are evenly coated.

7. Sprinkle the chopped walnuts over the top of the salad.

8. Serve the Roasted Beet and Arugula Salad immediately.

Nutritional Information (per serving):

- Carbs: 12 grams

- Fats: 11 grams

- Fiber: 3 grams

- Protein: 4 grams

Spinach and Strawberry Salad

Prep Time: 15 minutes
Cook Time: 0 minutes
Number of Servings: 4

Ingredients:

- 8 cups fresh baby spinach
- 2 cups fresh strawberries, hulled and sliced
- 1/4 cup sliced almonds
- 1/4 cup crumbled feta cheese
- 2 tablespoons extra-virgin olive oil
- 2 tablespoons balsamic vinegar
- 1/2 teaspoon honey
- 1/4 teaspoon salt
- 1/4 teaspoon black pepper

Instructions:

1. In a large salad bowl, add the fresh baby spinach, sliced strawberries, sliced almonds, and crumbled feta cheese.

2. In a small bowl, whisk the extra-virgin olive oil, balsamic vinegar, honey, salt, and black pepper to create the dressing.

3. Drizzle the dressing over the salad and toss gently to ensure the ingredients are evenly coated.

4. Serve the Spinach and Strawberry Salad immediately.

Nutritional Information (per serving):

- Carbs: 11 grams
- Fats: 8 grams
- Fiber: 3 grams

- Protein: 4 grams

Roasted Butternut Squash with Rosemary

Prep Time: 15 minutes
Cook Time: 30 minutes
Number of Servings: 4

Ingredients:

- 1 medium butternut squash, peeled, seeded, and diced into 1-inch cubes

- 2 tablespoons olive oil

- 2 teaspoons fresh rosemary, chopped

- 1/4 teaspoon salt

- 1/4 teaspoon black pepper

Instructions:

1. Preheat your oven to 400°F (200°C).

2. In a large mixing bowl, add the diced butternut squash with the olive oil, chopped rosemary, salt, and black pepper. Toss to ensure the squash cubes are evenly coated.

3. Spread the seasoned butternut squash cubes on a baking sheet in a single layer.

4. Roast in the preheated oven for about 30 minutes or until the squash is tender and lightly caramelized, flipping them halfway through the cooking time.

5. Once the butternut squash is roasted to your desired tenderness, take it out of the oven.

6. Serve the Roasted Butternut Squash with Rosemary hot.

Nutritional Information (per serving):

- Carbs: 22 grams

- Fats: 7 grams

- Fiber: 4 grams

- Protein: 1 gram

Brown Rice Pilaf with Cranberries and Almonds

Prep Time: 10 minutes
Cook Time: 45 minutes
Number of Servings: 4

Ingredients:

- 1 cup brown rice

- 2 cups low-sodium vegetable broth

- 1/4 cup dried cranberries

- 1/4 cup slivered almonds

- 1 small onion, finely chopped

- 1 clove garlic, minced

- 1 tablespoon olive oil

- 1/4 teaspoon salt

- 1/4 teaspoon black pepper

- 1/2 teaspoon dried thyme

Instructions:

1. In a large saucepan, heat the olive oil over medium heat. Add the finely chopped onion and sauté for about 3 minutes until translucent.

2. Add the minced garlic and continue to sauté for an additional minute until fragrant.

3. Stir in the brown rice and cook for 2-3 minutes, stirring frequently until the rice is lightly toasted.

4. Pour in the low-sodium vegetable broth, add the dried thyme, salt, and black pepper. Stir to combine.

5. Bring the mixture to a boil, then reduce the heat to low, cover the saucepan, and simmer for 45 minutes or until the rice is cooked and the liquid is absorbed.

6. Once the rice is cooked, take out the saucepan from the heat and let it sit, covered, for 5 minutes.

7. While the rice is resting, fluff it with a fork and stir in the dried cranberries and slivered almonds.

8. Serve the Brown Rice Pilaf with Cranberries and Almonds hot.

Nutritional Information (per serving):

- Carbs: 43 grams

- Fats: 8 grams

- Fiber: 4 grams

- Protein: 5 grams

Roasted Broccoli and Garlic

Prep Time: 10 minutes
Cook Time: 20 minutes
Number of Servings: 4

Ingredients:

- 1 pound fresh broccoli, trimmed into florets

- 4 cloves garlic, minced

- 2 tablespoons olive oil

- 1/4 teaspoon salt

- 1/4 teaspoon black pepper

Instructions:

1. Preheat your oven to 425°F (220°C).

2. In a large mixing bowl, add the trimmed broccoli florets, minced garlic, olive oil, salt, and black pepper. Toss to ensure the broccoli is evenly coated with the mixture.

3. Spread the seasoned broccoli out in a single layer on a baking sheet.

4. Roast in the preheated oven for about 20 minutes or until the broccoli is tender and slightly caramelized, stirring once or twice during roasting.

5. Once the broccoli is roasted to your desired tenderness, take it out of the oven.

6. Serve the Roasted Broccoli and Garlic hot.

Nutritional Information (per serving):

- Carbs: 6 grams

- Fats: 7 grams

- Fiber: 3 grams

- Protein: 2 grams

Spicy Cucumber Salad

Prep Time: 10 minutes
Cook Time: 0 minutes
Number of Servings: 4

Ingredients:

- 2 large cucumbers, thinly sliced

- 1/2 red onion, thinly sliced

- 2 tablespoons fresh cilantro, chopped

- 2 tablespoons rice vinegar

- 1 tablespoon olive oil

- 1/2 teaspoon red pepper flakes (adjust to taste)

- 1/4 teaspoon salt

- 1/4 teaspoon black pepper

Instructions:

1. In a large salad bowl, add the thinly sliced cucumbers and red onion.

2. In a small bowl, whisk the rice vinegar, olive oil, red pepper flakes, salt, and black pepper to create the dressing.

3. Drizzle the dressing over the cucumber and red onion slices.

4. Add the fresh chopped cilantro to the bowl.

5. Gently toss all the ingredients to ensure the cucumber and red onion are evenly coated with the dressing.

6. Refrigerate the salad for about 10-15 minutes to let the flavors meld.

7. Before serving, toss the salad once more to redistribute the dressing.

8. Serve the Spicy Cucumber Salad chilled.

Nutritional Information (per serving):

- Carbs: 8 grams

- Fats: 3 grams

- Fiber: 2 grams

- Protein: 1 gram

Quinoa Tabbouleh

Prep Time: 15 minutes
Cook Time: 15 minutes
Number of Servings: 4

Ingredients:

- 1 cup quinoa

- 2 cups water

- 2 cups fresh parsley, finely chopped

- 1 cup fresh mint, finely chopped

- 2 large tomatoes, diced

- 1/2 cucumber, diced

- 1/4 cup red onion, finely chopped

- 1/4 cup extra-virgin olive oil

- 1/4 cup lemon juice

- 2 cloves garlic, minced

- 1/4 teaspoon salt

- 1/4 teaspoon black pepper

Instructions:

1. Rinse the quinoa under cold water in a fine-mesh strainer. In a medium saucepan, add the rinsed quinoa and two cups of water. Bring to a boil, then reduce the heat to low, cover, and simmer for 15 minutes or until the quinoa is cooked and the liquid is absorbed. Take out from heat and let it cool.

2. In a large bowl, add the finely chopped fresh parsley and mint.

3. Add the diced tomatoes, cucumber, and finely chopped red onion to the bowl with the herbs.

4. In a separate small bowl, whisk the extra-virgin olive oil, lemon juice, minced garlic, salt, and black pepper to create the dressing.

5. Pour the dressing over the quinoa and toss to combine.

6. Gently fold the quinoa and dressing mixture into the bowl with the vegetables and herbs.

7. Serve the Quinoa Tabbouleh immediately or refrigerate until ready to serve.

Nutritional Information (per serving):

- Carbs: 32 grams

- Fats: 12 grams

- Fiber: 6 grams

- Protein: 6 grams

Balsamic Roasted Carrots

Prep Time: 10 minutes
Cook Time: 25 minutes
Number of Servings: 4

Ingredients:

- 1 pound fresh carrots, peeled and sliced into sticks

- 2 tablespoons olive oil

- 2 tablespoons balsamic vinegar

- 2 cloves garlic, minced

- 1/4 teaspoon salt

- 1/4 teaspoon black pepper

- 2 tablespoons fresh parsley, chopped (for garnish)

Instructions:

1. Preheat your oven to 425°F (220°C).

2. In a mixing bowl, add the sliced carrot sticks, olive oil, balsamic vinegar, minced garlic, salt, and black pepper. Toss to ensure the carrots are evenly coated.

3. Spread the seasoned carrot sticks out in a single layer on a baking sheet.

4. Roast in the preheated oven for 20-25 minutes or until the carrots are tender and slightly caramelized, stirring once or twice during roasting.

5. Once the carrots are roasted to your desired tenderness, take them out of the oven.

6. Garnish with fresh chopped parsley before serving.

Nutritional Information (per serving):

- Carbs: 10 grams

- Fats: 7 grams

- Fiber: 3 grams

- Protein: 1 gram

Garlic Parmesan Mashed Cauliflower

Prep Time: 10 minutes
Cook Time: 15 minutes
Number of Servings: 4

Ingredients:

- 1 large head of cauliflower, cut into florets

- 2 cloves garlic, minced

- 2 tablespoons grated Parmesan cheese

- 1/4 cup low-sodium chicken or vegetable broth

- 2 tablespoons low-fat milk

- 1/4 teaspoon salt

- 1/4 teaspoon black pepper

- 1 tablespoon fresh chives, chopped (for garnish)

Instructions:

1. Steam the cauliflower florets until they are tender, about 10-12 minutes.

2. In a food processor, add the steamed cauliflower, minced garlic, grated Parmesan cheese, low-sodium chicken or vegetable broth, low-fat milk, salt, and black pepper.

3. Process the mixture until it reaches a smooth and creamy consistency.

4. If the mixture is too thick, you can add a little more broth or milk to achieve your desired consistency.

5. Transfer the mashed cauliflower to a serving bowl.

6. Garnish with fresh chopped chives before serving.

Nutritional Information (per serving):

- Carbs: 7 grams

- Fats: 2 grams

- Fiber: 3 grams

- Protein: 4 grams

Lemon Herb Quinoa Pilaf

Prep Time: 15 minutes
Cook Time: 15 minutes
Number of Servings: 4

Ingredients:

- 1 cup quinoa
- 2 cups low-sodium vegetable broth
- 2 tablespoons fresh parsley, chopped
- 2 tablespoons fresh chives, chopped
- 1 tablespoon fresh dill, chopped
- 2 tablespoons lemon juice
- 2 tablespoons extra-virgin olive oil
- 1/4 teaspoon salt
- 1/4 teaspoon black pepper
- 1/4 cup slivered almonds (for garnish)

Instructions:

1. Rinse the quinoa under cold water in a fine-mesh strainer. In a medium saucepan, add the rinsed quinoa and two cups of low-sodium vegetable broth. Bring to a boil, then reduce the heat to low, cover, and simmer for 15 minutes or until the quinoa is cooked and the liquid is absorbed. Take out from heat and let it cool.

2. In a large mixing bowl, add the chopped fresh parsley, chives, and dill.

3. In a separate small bowl, whisk the lemon juice, extra-virgin olive oil, salt, and black pepper to create the dressing.

4. Fluff the cooked quinoa with a fork and add it to the bowl with the herbs.

5. Pour the dressing over the quinoa and herbs, then toss to combine.

6. Garnish with slivered almonds before serving.

Nutritional Information (per serving):

- Carbs: 32 grams

- Fats: 9 grams

- Fiber: 3 grams

- Protein: 6 grams

Sauteed Spinach with Pine Nuts

Prep Time: 5 minutes
Cook Time: 5 minutes
Number of Servings: 4

Ingredients:

- 1 pound fresh spinach

- 2 tablespoons olive oil

- 2 cloves garlic, minced

- 1/4 cup pine nuts

- 1/4 teaspoon salt

- 1/4 teaspoon black pepper

- 1/2 teaspoon lemon zest (for garnish)

Instructions:

1. Wash the fresh spinach and Take out any tough stems.

2. In a large skillet, heat the olive oil over medium heat.

3. Add the minced garlic and pine nuts to the skillet. Saute for about 1-2 minutes until the garlic is fragrant and the pine nuts are lightly toasted.

4. Add the fresh spinach to the skillet. Use tongs or a spatula to toss and stir the spinach as it wilts. This should take about 2-3 minutes.

5. Season the sauteed spinach with salt and black pepper. Toss to combine.

6. Transfer the sauteed spinach and pine nuts to a serving dish.

7. Garnish with lemon zest before serving.

Nutritional Information (per serving):

- Carbs: 3 grams

- Fats: 7 grams

- Fiber: 2 grams

- Protein: 3 grams

Roasted Brussels Sprouts with Cranberries

Prep Time: 10 minutes
Cook Time: 25 minutes
Number of Servings: 4

Ingredients:

- 1 pound fresh Brussels sprouts, trimmed and halved

- 1/2 cup fresh cranberries

- 2 tablespoons olive oil

- 2 tablespoons balsamic vinegar

- 1 tablespoon honey

- 1/4 teaspoon salt

- 1/4 teaspoon black pepper

- 2 tablespoons chopped pecans (for garnish)

Instructions:

1. Preheat your oven to 425°F (220°C).

2. In a large mixing bowl, add the trimmed and halved Brussels sprouts, fresh cranberries, olive oil, balsamic vinegar, honey, salt, and black pepper. Toss to ensure the Brussels sprouts and cranberries are evenly coated.

3. Spread the seasoned Brussels sprouts and cranberries on a baking sheet in a single layer.

4. Roast in the preheated oven for about 25 minutes or until the Brussels sprouts are tender and slightly caramelized, stirring once during roasting.

5. Once the Brussels sprouts are roasted to your desired tenderness, take them out of the oven.

6. Garnish with chopped pecans before serving.

Nutritional Information (per serving):

- Carbs: 20 grams

- Fats: 7 grams

- Fiber: 5 grams

- Protein: 3 grams

Chapter 8: Desserts

Mixed Berry Parfait

Prep Time: 15 minutes
Cook Time: 0 minutes
Number of Servings: 4

Ingredients:

- 2 cups fresh mixed berries (strawberries, blueberries, raspberries)

- 1 cup low-fat Greek yogurt

- 1/2 cup rolled oats

- 1/4 cup chopped almonds

- 2 tablespoons honey

- 1 teaspoon vanilla extract

Instructions:

1. In a mixing bowl, add one cup of low-fat Greek yogurt with one teaspoon of vanilla extract. Stir until well blended.

2. In a separate bowl, add two cups of fresh mixed berries (strawberries, blueberries, raspberries). If needed, you can slice the strawberries into bite-sized pieces.

3. In a dry skillet over low heat, toast 1/2 cup of rolled oats and 1/4 cup of chopped almonds until they turn golden and fragrant, about 2-3 minutes. Stir frequently to avoid burning.

4. To assemble the parfaits, take four serving glasses or bowls. Start by adding a layer of the yogurt mixture at the bottom of each glass.

5. Add a layer of the mixed berries on top of the yogurt.

6. Sprinkle the toasted oats and almonds mixture evenly over the berries.

7. Drizzle two tablespoons of honey evenly over each parfait.

8. Repeat the layers until the glasses are filled, finishing with a layer of mixed berries on top.

9. Serve immediately or refrigerate for later consumption.

Nutritional Information (per serving):

- Carbs: 38 grams

- Fats: 7 grams

- Fiber: 6 grams

- Protein: 8 grams

Dark Chocolate-Dipped Strawberries
Prep Time: 15 minutes
Cook Time: 5 minutes
Number of Servings: 4

Ingredients:

- 1 pint fresh strawberries

- 4 ounces dark chocolate (70% cocoa or higher)

- 1 tablespoon unsalted butter

- 1 teaspoon vanilla extract

- 2 tablespoons chopped nuts (e.g., almonds or walnuts)

- 1 tablespoon shredded coconut (unsweetened)

- 1 teaspoon honey

Instructions:

1. Wash and thoroughly dry 1 pint of fresh strawberries. Ensure they are completely dry to help the chocolate adhere.

2. In a small saucepan, melt 4 ounces of dark chocolate and one tablespoon of unsalted butter over low heat. Stir frequently until smooth. Once melted, stir in one teaspoon of vanilla extract.

3. Prepare a baking sheet with parchment paper.

4. Hold each strawberry by the stem, dip it into the melted dark chocolate, and twirl it to coat evenly. Allow any excess chocolate to drip back into the saucepan.

5. Place each chocolate-dipped strawberry on the prepared baking sheet.

6. While the chocolate is still wet, sprinkle two tablespoons of chopped nuts and one tablespoon of shredded coconut evenly over the strawberries.

7. Drizzle one teaspoon of honey over the strawberries.

8. Allow the chocolate to cool and harden. You can speed up the process by placing the baking sheet in the refrigerator for about 30 minutes.

9. Once the chocolate is firm, serve and enjoy.

Nutritional Information (per serving):

- Carbs: 20 grams

- Fats: 12 grams

- Fiber: 4 grams

- Protein: 3 grams

Greek Yogurt with Honey and Nuts

Prep Time: 5 minutes
Cook Time: 0 minutes
Number of Servings: 4

Ingredients:

- 2 cups low-fat Greek yogurt

- 4 tablespoons honey

- 1/2 cup chopped nuts (e.g., almonds, walnuts)

- 1 teaspoon vanilla extract

Instructions:

1. In a mixing bowl, add two cups of low-fat Greek yogurt with one teaspoon of vanilla extract. Stir until well blended.

2. Divide the vanilla-infused Greek yogurt equally among four serving bowls.

3. Drizzle one tablespoon of honey over the yogurt in each bowl.

4. Sprinkle two tablespoons of chopped nuts (e.g., almonds, walnuts) evenly over each serving.

5. Serve immediately or refrigerate for later.

Nutritional Information (per serving):

- Carbs: 17 grams

- Fats: 8 grams

- Fiber: 1 gram

- Protein: 15 grams

Baked Apples with Cinnamon

Prep Time: 15 minutes
Cook Time: 30 minutes
Number of Servings: 4

Ingredients:

- 4 medium-sized apples

- 2 tablespoons honey

- 1/2 teaspoon ground cinnamon

- 1/4 cup chopped nuts (e.g., almonds, pecans)

- 1 tablespoon unsalted butter

Instructions:

1. Preheat your oven to 375°F (190°C).

2. Wash and core 4 medium-sized apples, leaving the bottom intact to create a well for the filling. You can peel them if preferred, but leaving the skin on provides extra fiber.

3. In a small bowl, mix two tablespoons of honey with 1/2 teaspoon of ground cinnamon to create a cinnamon-honey glaze.

4. Place the cored apples in a baking dish.

5. Spoon the cinnamon-honey glaze evenly into the wells of the apples.

6. Divide 1/4 cup of chopped nuts (e.g., almonds, pecans) among the apples, filling the wells.

7. Top each apple with a 1/4 tablespoon of unsalted butter.

8. Cover the baking dish with foil and bake in the preheated oven for approximately 25-30 minutes or until the apples are tender.

9. Take out the foil and bake for an additional 5 minutes to allow the tops to caramelize.

10. Serve the baked apples warm, optionally with a dollop of Greek yogurt or a sprinkle of extra cinnamon.

Nutritional Information (per serving):

- Carbs: 29 grams

- Fats: 8 grams

- Fiber: 5 grams

- Protein: 2 grams

Mango Sorbet

Prep Time: 10 minutes
Cook Time: 0 minutes
Number of Servings: 4

Ingredients:

- 4 cups diced fresh mango (about 4-5 medium-sized mangoes)
- 1/4 cup honey
- 1 tablespoon fresh lime juice
- 1/4 cup water

Instructions:

1. Start by peeling, pitting, and dicing 4 cups of fresh mangoes. Ensure they are ripe and sweet for the best flavor.

2. Place the diced mangoes in a single layer on a baking sheet lined with parchment paper. Freeze for at least 2 hours or until the mango pieces are solid.

3. In a blender or food processor, add the frozen mango chunks, 1/4 cup of honey, one tablespoon of fresh lime juice, and 1/4 cup of water.

4. Blend the mixture until it becomes smooth and creamy, scraping down the sides as needed. If the sorbet is too thick, you can add a little more water, one tablespoon at a time, to help with blending.

5. Once the sorbet is well-blended, transfer it to an airtight container and freeze for an additional 1-2 hours to firm it up slightly.

6. Before serving, allow the sorbet to sit at room temperature for a few minutes to soften for easier scooping.

7. Scoop the mango sorbet into bowls or cones and serve.

Nutritional Information (per serving):

- Carbs: 36 grams

- Fats: 1 gram

- Fiber: 3 grams

- Protein: 1 gram

Chia Seed Pudding with Berries

Prep Time: 5 minutes (plus chilling time)
Cook Time: 0 minutes
Number of Servings: 4

Ingredients:

- 1 cup unsweetened almond milk

- 1/4 cup chia seeds

- 2 tablespoons honey

- 1 teaspoon vanilla extract

- 1 cup mixed berries (strawberries, blueberries, raspberries)

Instructions:

1. In a mixing bowl, add one cup of unsweetened almond milk, 1/4 cup of chia seeds, two tablespoons of honey, and one teaspoon of vanilla extract. Stir the mixture well to ensure the chia seeds are evenly distributed.

2. Cover the bowl and refrigerate for at least 4 hours or overnight, allowing the chia seeds to absorb the liquid and create a pudding-like consistency. Be sure to stir it a couple of times during the first hour to prevent clumping.

3. Before serving, wash and prepare one cup of mixed berries, which can include strawberries, blueberries, and raspberries. If necessary, slice the strawberries into smaller pieces.

4. Divide the chia seed pudding mixture into four serving bowls.

5. Top each serving with a quarter of the mixed berries.

6. Drizzle a little extra honey on top if desired.

7. Serve your Chia Seed Pudding with Berries as a nutritious and delicious breakfast or snack.

Nutritional Information (per serving):

- Carbs: 24 grams

- Fats: 7 grams

- Fiber: 9 grams

- Protein: 5 grams

Banana and Almond Butter Bites

Prep Time: 10 minutes
Cook Time: 0 minutes
Number of Servings: 4

Ingredients:

- 2 large bananas

- 1/4 cup natural almond butter

- 1/4 teaspoon ground cinnamon

- 2 tablespoons chopped almonds

- 2 tablespoons dried cranberries (unsweetened)

Instructions:

1. Start by peeling and slicing 2 large bananas into 1/2-inch thick rounds.

2. In a small bowl, mix 1/4 cup of natural almond butter with 1/4 teaspoon of ground cinnamon.

3. Spread a small amount of the almond butter mixture onto each banana slice.

4. Sprinkle two tablespoons of chopped almonds and two tablespoons of dried cranberries evenly over the almond butter-coated banana slices.

5. Serve your Banana and Almond Butter Bites immediately as a wholesome and delicious snack.

Nutritional Information (per serving):

- Carbs: 24 grams

- Fats: 11 grams

- Fiber: 4 grams

- Protein: 5 grams

Poached Pears in Red Wine

Prep Time: 15 minutes
Cook Time: 30 minutes
Number of Servings: 4

Ingredients:

- 4 ripe but firm pears

- 1 bottle (750ml) of red wine (choose a dry red wine)

- 1/2 cup honey

- 1 cinnamon stick

- 4 whole cloves

- 1 orange, zested and juiced

Instructions:

1. Peel the pears, leaving the stem intact. If desired, you can also cut a thin slice off the bottom of each pear to ensure they stand upright in the pot.

2. In a large saucepan or pot, add the red wine, 1/2 cup of honey, the zest and juice of one orange, 1 cinnamon stick, and 4 whole cloves. Stir sufficiently.

3. Place the pears in the red wine mixture, ensuring they are fully submerged. If necessary, add a little water to cover them.

4. Bring the mixture to a gentle simmer over medium heat.

5. Once simmering, reduce the heat to low, cover, and let the pears poach for about 20-30 minutes. The pears should be tender but not too soft. Test by gently piercing them with a fork.

6. Carefully take out the poached pears from the red wine mixture and set them aside on a plate.

7. Continue simmering the red wine mixture uncovered for about 10-15 minutes or until it reduces and thickens into a syrupy consistency.

8. Pour the red wine syrup over the poached pears.

9. Serve your Poached Pears in Red Wine as a delightful and elegant dessert.

Nutritional Information (per serving):

- Carbs: 50 grams

- Fats: 0 grams

- Fiber: 6 grams

- Protein: 1 gram

Chocolate Avocado Mousse

Prep Time: 10 minutes
Cook Time: 0 minutes
Number of Servings: 4

Ingredients:

- 2 ripe avocados

- 1/4 cup unsweetened cocoa powder

- 1/4 cup honey

- 1 teaspoon vanilla extract

- 1/4 cup unsweetened almond milk

- A pinch of salt

Instructions:

1. Cut 2 ripe avocados in half, take out the pits, and scoop the flesh into a food processor.

2. Add 1/4 cup of unsweetened cocoa powder, 1/4 cup of honey, one teaspoon of vanilla extract, and a pinch of salt to the avocados.

3. Blend the mixture until smooth, scraping down the sides of the food processor as needed to ensure it's well mixed.

4. While the food processor is running, slowly add 1/4 cup of unsweetened almond milk to the mixture. Continue blending until you achieve a creamy and mousse-like consistency.

5. Taste the mousse and adjust the sweetness with more honey if needed.

6. Divide the Chocolate Avocado Mousse into four serving bowls.

7. Refrigerate for at least 30 minutes to chill and set.

8. Serve your Chocolate Avocado Mousse as a delicious and healthy dessert.

Nutritional Information (per serving):

- Carbs: 24 grams

- Fats: 11 grams

- Fiber: 6 grams

- Protein: 2 grams

Pineapple and Mint Sorbet

Prep Time: 10 minutes (plus freezing time)
Cook Time: 0 minutes
Number of Servings: 4

Ingredients:

- 4 cups fresh pineapple chunks

- 1/4 cup honey

- 1/4 cup fresh mint leaves

- 1 tablespoon fresh lime juice

- 1/4 cup water

Instructions:

1. Start by preparing 4 cups of fresh pineapple chunks. You can use a fresh pineapple and cut it into chunks, or use pre-cut pineapple.

2. In a blender or food processor, add the pineapple chunks, 1/4 cup of honey, 1/4 cup of fresh mint leaves, one tablespoon of fresh lime juice, and 1/4 cup of water.

3. Blend the mixture until it's smooth and well combined.

4. Taste the mixture and adjust the sweetness or lime flavor according to your preference, adding more honey or lime juice if needed.

5. Pour the pineapple and mint mixture into a shallow container and cover it.

6. Place the container in the freezer and let it freeze for at least 4-6 hours, or until the sorbet is firm.

7. Before serving, allow the sorbet to sit at room temperature for a few minutes to soften for easier scooping.

8. Serve your Pineapple and Mint Sorbet as a refreshing and healthy dessert.

Nutritional Information (per serving):

- Carbs: 34 grams

- Fats: 0 grams

- Fiber: 2 grams

- Protein: 1 gram

Cinnamon Baked Peaches

Prep Time: 10 minutes
Cook Time: 25 minutes
Number of Servings: 4

Ingredients:

- 4 ripe but firm peaches

- 2 tablespoons honey

- 1/2 teaspoon ground cinnamon

- 1/4 cup chopped nuts (e.g., almonds, walnuts)

- 1/4 cup low-fat Greek yogurt (for serving)

Instructions:

1. Preheat your oven to 350°F (175°C).

2. Cut 4 ripe but firm peaches in half and take out the pits. Place them in a baking dish with the cut side facing up.

3. Drizzle two tablespoons of honey evenly over the peaches.

4. In a small bowl, mix 1/2 teaspoon of ground cinnamon with 1/4 cup of chopped nuts (e.g., almonds, walnuts).

5. Sprinkle the cinnamon and nut mixture over the honey-drizzled peaches.

6. Bake the peaches in the preheated oven for about 20-25 minutes, or until they are tender and caramelized.

7. While the peaches are baking, you can prepare 1/4 cup of low-fat Greek yogurt for serving.

8. Serve the warm Cinnamon Baked Peaches with a dollop of Greek yogurt on top as a delicious and healthy dessert.

Nutritional Information (per serving):

- Carbs: 23 grams
- Fats: 6 grams
- Fiber: 3 grams
- Protein: 4 grams

Almond and Coconut Energy Balls

Prep Time: 15 minutes
Cook Time: 0 minutes
Number of Servings: 12

Ingredients:

- 1 cup rolled oats
- 1/2 cup unsweetened almond butter
- 1/4 cup honey
- 1/4 cup shredded unsweetened coconut
- 1/4 cup chopped almonds
- 1/4 cup chopped dates
- 1/2 teaspoon vanilla extract
- A pinch of salt

Instructions:

1. In a large mixing bowl, add one cup of rolled oats, 1/2 cup of unsweetened almond butter, 1/4 cup of honey, 1/4 cup of shredded unsweetened coconut, 1/4 cup of chopped almonds, 1/4 cup of chopped dates, 1/2 teaspoon of vanilla extract, and a pinch of salt.

2. Stir the mixture thoroughly until all the ingredients are well combined. The mixture should be sticky and easy to shape.

3. Take small portions of the mixture and roll them into 12 individual balls.

4. Place the energy balls on a plate or tray and refrigerate for about 30 minutes to help them set.

5. Once chilled and firm, your Almond and Coconut Energy Balls are ready to be served.

Nutritional Information (per serving - 1 ball):

-   Carbs: 18 grams

-   Fats: 9 grams

-   Fiber: 2 grams

-   Protein: 4 grams

Raspberry Frozen Yogurt

Prep Time: 10 minutes (plus freezing time)
Cook Time: 0 minutes
Number of Servings: 4

Ingredients:

-   3 cups frozen raspberries

-   1/4 cup honey

-   2 cups low-fat Greek yogurt

- 1 teaspoon vanilla extract

- Fresh mint leaves for garnish (optional)

Instructions:

1. In a blender or food processor, add three cups of frozen raspberries.

2. Add 1/4 cup of honey to the raspberries.

3. Add two cups of low-fat Greek yogurt and one teaspoon of vanilla extract to the blender as well.

4. Blend the mixture until it becomes smooth and creamy, scraping down the sides of the blender as needed to ensure it's well mixed.

5. Taste the frozen yogurt and adjust the sweetness with more honey if needed.

6. Pour the raspberry frozen yogurt mixture into a lidded container.

7. Place the container in the freezer and let it freeze for at least 4-6 hours, or until the frozen yogurt is firm.

8. Before serving, allow the frozen yogurt to sit at room temperature for a few minutes to soften for easier scooping.

9. Garnish with fresh mint leaves if desired and serve your Raspberry Frozen Yogurt as a delightful and heart-healthy dessert.

Nutritional Information (per serving):

- Carbs: 33 grams

- Fats: 1 gram

- Fiber: 6 grams

- Protein: 7 grams

Oatmeal Raisin Cookies

Prep Time: 15 minutes
Cook Time: 12-15 minutes
Number of Servings: 24

Ingredients:

- 1 cup whole wheat flour

- 1 cup rolled oats

- 1/2 teaspoon baking soda

- 1/2 teaspoon ground cinnamon

- 1/4 teaspoon salt

- 1/2 cup unsalted butter, softened

- 1/2 cup honey

- 1 large egg

- 1 teaspoon vanilla extract

- 1 cup raisins

Instructions:

1. Preheat your oven to 350°F (175°C).

2. In a mixing bowl, add one cup of whole wheat flour, one cup of rolled oats, 1/2 teaspoon of baking soda, 1/2 teaspoon of ground cinnamon, and 1/4 teaspoon of salt. Mix sufficiently and set aside.

3. In an extra bowl, cream together 1/2 cup of softened unsalted butter and 1/2 cup of honey until the mixture is light and fluffy.

4. Beat in 1 large egg and one teaspoon of vanilla extract.

5. Gradually add the dry ingredient mixture to the wet ingredients, stirring until just combined.

6. Fold in one cup of raisins.

7. Drop rounded tablespoons of the cookie dough onto ungreased baking sheets, spacing them about 2 inches apart.

8. Bake in the preheated oven for 12-15 minutes, or until the cookies are golden brown around the edges.

9. Allow the cookies to cool on the baking sheets for a few minutes, then transfer them to wire racks to cool completely, and then serve.

Nutritional Information (per serving - 1 cookie):

- Carbs: 15 grams

- Fats: 5 grams

- Fiber: 1.5 grams

- Protein: 1 gram

Honey and Walnut Baked Pears
Prep Time: 10 minutes
Cook Time: 30 minutes
Number of Servings: 4

Ingredients:

- 4 ripe but firm pears

- 1/4 cup honey

- 1/2 cup chopped walnuts

- 1/2 teaspoon ground cinnamon

- 1/4 cup low-fat Greek yogurt (for serving)

Instructions:

1. Preheat your oven to 375°F (190°C).

2. Cut 4 ripe but firm pears in half and take out the cores, leaving a small well for the filling. You can also slice a thin piece off the bottom of each pear to help them stand upright in the baking dish.

3. Drizzle 1/4 cup of honey evenly over the pear halves.

4. In a small bowl, add 1/2 cup of chopped walnuts and 1/2 teaspoon of ground cinnamon. Mix sufficiently.

5. Sprinkle the walnut and cinnamon mixture evenly over the honey-drizzled pears.

6. Place the pear halves in a baking dish and add about 1/4 inch of water to the bottom of the dish.

7. Cover the baking dish with aluminum foil and bake in the preheated oven for about 20-25 minutes, or until the pears are tender.

8. Take out the foil and bake for an additional 5-10 minutes to allow the tops to caramelize slightly.

9. Serve your Honey and Walnut Baked Pears warm, with a dollop of low-fat Greek yogurt on top, as a heart-healthy and delicious dessert.

Nutritional Information (per serving):

- Carbs: 25 grams

- Fats: 9 grams

- Fiber: 5 grams

- Protein: 3 grams

Berry and Yogurt Parfait with Granola

Prep Time: 10 minutes
Cook Time: 0 minutes
Number of Servings: 4

Ingredients:

- 2 cups low-fat Greek yogurt

- 2 cups mixed berries (strawberries, blueberries, raspberries)

- 1/2 cup granola (low-sugar, high-fiber)

- 2 tablespoons honey

- 1/4 cup chopped almonds (optional)

Instructions:

1. In four serving glasses or bowls, start by layering 1/4 cup of low-fat Greek yogurt in the bottom of each.

2. Add 1/4 cup of mixed berries (strawberries, blueberries, raspberries) on top of the yogurt in each glass.

3. Sprinkle two tablespoons of granola (low-sugar, high-fiber) over the berries in each glass.

4. Drizzle 1/2 tablespoon of honey over the granola in each glass.

5. If desired, add one tablespoon of chopped almonds on top of the honey in each glass.

6. Repeat these layers one more time for each glass, starting with 1/4 cup of low-fat Greek yogurt and finishing with one tablespoon of chopped almonds (if using).

7. Serve your Berry and Yogurt Parfait with Granola as a satisfying and heart-healthy breakfast or snack.

Nutritional Information (per serving):

- Carbs: 35 grams

- Fats: 9 grams

- Fiber: 6 grams

- Protein: 11 grams

Dark Chocolate-Covered Banana Bites

Prep Time: 15 minutes (plus freezing time)
Cook Time: 0 minutes
Number of Servings: 4

Ingredients:

- 2 large bananas

- 4 ounces dark chocolate (70% cocoa or higher)

- 2 tablespoons unsweetened almond butter

- 1/4 cup chopped nuts (e.g., almonds, walnuts)

- 1/4 cup unsweetened shredded coconut

Instructions:

1. Begin by peeling and slicing 2 large bananas into 1/2-inch thick rounds.

2. In a microwave-safe bowl, break 4 ounces of dark chocolate (70% cocoa or higher) into small pieces. Add two tablespoons of unsweetened almond butter to the bowl as well.

3. Microwave the chocolate and almond butter in 20-30 second intervals, stirring each time until the mixture is smooth and fully melted.

4. Line a tray or plate with parchment paper.

5. Dip each banana slice into the dark chocolate-almond butter mixture, ensuring they are well-coated. Place them on the parchment paper.

6. Sprinkle 1/4 cup of chopped nuts (e.g., almonds, walnuts) and 1/4 cup of unsweetened shredded coconut over the banana slices.

7. Place the tray or plate in the freezer and let the banana bites freeze for at least 2 hours, or until the chocolate is completely set.

8. Serve your Dark Chocolate-Covered Banana Bites as a heart-healthy and indulgent dessert or snack.

Nutritional Information (per serving):

- Carbs: 25 grams

- Fats: 16 grams

- Fiber: 5 grams

- Protein: 4 grams

Chia Seed Chocolate Pudding

Prep Time: 10 minutes (plus chilling time)
Cook Time: 0 minutes
Number of Servings: 4

Ingredients:

- 1/2 cup chia seeds

- 2 cups unsweetened almond milk

- 1/4 cup unsweetened cocoa powder

- 1/4 cup honey

- 1 teaspoon vanilla extract

- A pinch of salt

Instructions:

1. In a mixing bowl, add 1/2 cup of chia seeds and two cups of unsweetened almond milk. Stir sufficiently to ensure the chia seeds are evenly distributed in the almond milk.

2. Add 1/4 cup of unsweetened cocoa powder to the mixture. Stir until the cocoa powder is fully incorporated.

3. Mix in 1/4 cup of honey, one teaspoon of vanilla extract, and a pinch of salt. Continue to stir until all ingredients are well combined.

4. Cover the bowl and refrigerate for at least 2-3 hours, or overnight. This will allow the chia seeds to absorb the liquid and create a pudding-like consistency.

5. Before serving, give the Chia Seed Chocolate Pudding a good stir to readd any settled ingredients.

6. Serve your Chia Seed Chocolate Pudding as a heart-healthy and satisfying dessert.

Nutritional Information (per serving):

- Carbs: 21 grams

- Fats: 7 grams

- Fiber: 11 grams

- Protein: 4 grams

Almond and Date Energy Bars

Prep Time: 15 minutes
Cook Time: 0 minutes
Number of Servings: 12

Ingredients:

- 1 cup rolled oats

- 1/2 cup almonds, finely chopped

- 1/2 cup dates, pitted and finely chopped

- 1/4 cup unsweetened almond butter

- 2 tablespoons honey

- 1/2 teaspoon vanilla extract

- A pinch of salt

- 1/4 cup dried cranberries (optional)

Instructions:

1. In a large mixing bowl, add one cup of rolled oats, 1/2 cup of finely chopped almonds, and 1/2 cup of finely chopped dates. If you're using dried cranberries, add them now.

2. In a separate microwave-safe bowl, heat 1/4 cup of unsweetened almond butter and two tablespoons of honey until they are soft and easy to mix. This should take about 20-30 seconds in the microwave.

3. Stir 1/2 teaspoon of vanilla extract and a pinch of salt into the almond butter and honey mixture.

4. Pour the almond butter mixture over the dry ingredients in the large mixing bowl.

5. Mix everything together until the ingredients are well combined and the mixture becomes sticky and clumps together.

6. Line a 9x9-inch (23x23 cm) square baking pan with parchment paper.

7. Transfer the mixture into the lined pan and press it down firmly to create an even layer.

8. Refrigerate for at least 2 hours to allow the bars to set.

9. Once chilled, Take out from the pan and cut into 12 bars.

10. Serve your Almond and Date Energy Bars as a satisfying and heart-healthy snack.

Nutritional Information (per serving):

- Carbs: 25 grams

- Fats: 7 grams

- Fiber: 3 grams

- Protein: 4 grams

Mango and Lime Sorbet

Prep Time: 10 minutes (plus freezing time)
Cook Time: 0 minutes
Number of Servings: 4

Ingredients:

- 4 cups frozen mango chunks

- 1/4 cup freshly squeezed lime juice

- 2 tablespoons honey

- Zest of one lime

- Fresh mint leaves for garnish (optional)

Instructions:

1. In a blender or food processor, add 4 cups of frozen mango chunks.

2. Squeeze the juice of fresh limes to obtain 1/4 cup of lime juice.

3. Add the freshly squeezed lime juice to the blender with the mango chunks.

4. Zest one lime and add the zest to the blender as well.

5. Pour two tablespoons of honey into the blender.

6. Blend the mixture until it's smooth and well combined.

7. Taste the sorbet mixture and adjust the sweetness or lime flavor according to your preference, adding more honey or lime juice if needed.

8. Pour the mango and lime sorbet mixture into a shallow container and cover it.

9. Place the container in the freezer and let it freeze for at least 4-6 hours, or until the sorbet is firm.

10. Before serving, allow the sorbet to sit at room temperature for a few minutes to soften for easier scooping.

11. Garnish with fresh mint leaves if desired and serve your Mango and Lime Sorbet as a refreshing and heart-healthy dessert.

Nutritional Information (per serving):

- Carbs: 45 grams

- Fats: 1 gram

- Fiber: 4 grams

- Protein: 1 gram

Baked Cinnamon Apples with Walnuts

Prep Time: 15 minutes
Cook Time: 30 minutes
Number of Servings: 4

Ingredients:

- 4 large apples, cored and sliced

- 1/4 cup chopped walnuts

- 2 tablespoons honey

- 1/2 teaspoon ground cinnamon

- 1/4 teaspoon vanilla extract

- A pinch of salt

- 1/4 cup low-fat Greek yogurt (for serving)

Instructions:

1. Preheat your oven to 375°F (190°C).

2. Core and slice 4 large apples, keeping the peel on, and place them in a baking dish.

3. In a small bowl, add 1/4 cup of chopped walnuts, two tablespoons of honey, 1/2 teaspoon of ground cinnamon, 1/4 teaspoon of vanilla extract, and a pinch of salt. Mix sufficiently.

4. Drizzle the honey and walnut mixture over the sliced apples in the baking dish.

5. Toss the apples to ensure they are evenly coated with the honey and walnut mixture.

6. Cover the baking dish with aluminum foil and bake in the preheated oven for about 20 minutes.

7. Take out the foil and bake for an additional 10-15 minutes or until the apples are tender and slightly caramelized.

8. Serve the Baked Cinnamon Apples with Walnuts warm, with a dollop of low-fat Greek yogurt on top, as a heart-healthy and satisfying dessert.

Nutritional Information (per serving):

- Carbs: 30 grams

- Fats: 6 grams

- Fiber: 5 grams

- Protein: 3 grams

Greek Yogurt with Honey and Pistachios

Prep Time: 5 minutes
Cook Time: 0 minutes
Number of Servings: 2

Ingredients:

- 2 cups low-fat Greek yogurt

- 2 tablespoons honey

- 1/4 cup unsalted pistachios, chopped

Instructions:

1. In a bowl, divide two cups of low-fat Greek yogurt evenly into two serving dishes.

2. Drizzle two tablespoons of honey over each portion of Greek yogurt.

3. Sprinkle 1/8 cup (which is two tablespoons) of chopped unsalted pistachios over each serving.

4. Serve your Greek Yogurt with Honey and Pistachios immediately as a heart-healthy and delightful dessert or snack.

Nutritional Information (per serving):

- Carbs: 32 grams

- Fats: 12 grams

- Fiber: 3 grams

- Protein: 15 grams

Lemon Coconut Bliss Balls

Prep Time: 15 minutes
Cook Time: 0 minutes
Number of Servings: 12

Ingredients:

- 1 cup rolled oats

- 1/2 cup unsweetened shredded coconut

- Zest of 1 lemon

- 2 tablespoons fresh lemon juice

- 1/4 cup honey

- 1/4 cup almond butter

- 1/4 teaspoon vanilla extract

- A pinch of salt

Instructions:

1. In a food processor, add one cup of rolled oats, 1/2 cup of unsweetened shredded coconut, and the zest of 1 lemon.

2. Process the mixture until the oats are finely ground and everything is well combined.

3. Add two tablespoons of fresh lemon juice, 1/4 cup of honey, 1/4 cup of almond butter, 1/4 teaspoon of vanilla extract, and a pinch of salt to the food processor.

4. Process the mixture again until it forms a sticky, dough-like consistency.

5. Scoop out small portions of the mixture and roll them into 12 bite-sized balls.

6. Place the Lemon Coconut Bliss Balls on a tray or plate lined with parchment paper.

7. Refrigerate the bliss balls for at least 30 minutes to allow them to set.

8. Serve your Lemon Coconut Bliss Balls as a heart-healthy and energizing snack or dessert.

Nutritional Information (per serving - 1 ball):

- Carbs: 16 grams

- Fats: 6 grams

- Fiber: 2 grams

- Protein: 3 grams

Chapter 9: Weekly Meal Plan & Meal Planning Preparation

Meal planning involves the process of organizing and preparing meals in advance. Efficient meal planning and preparation are important for successfully incorporating the DASH Diet into your lifestyle. This chapter provides you with the tools and strategies necessary to make your culinary endeavors more efficient, so that every meal you prepare follows the heart-healthy principles of the DASH Diet.

Weekly Meal Planning Guide

Start your DASH Diet journey by creating a well-planned weekly meal plan. This cookbook offers a 30-day diverse meal plan comprising breakfasts, lunches, dinners, and snacks to help you begin your DASH diet journey on a strong footing. Aim to include a mix of whole grains, lean proteins, fruits, and vegetables in every meal. This guide will help you prepare a week's worth of tasty and varied meals in addition to making your grocery shopping easier.

8-Week DASH Diet Meal Plan

Week 1:

Day 1:

- **Breakfast:** Greek Yogurt Parfait with Honey and Berries
- **Lunch:** Chickpea and Spinach Dip with Sliced Cucumbers
- **Dinner:** Grilled Lemon Herb Chicken with Roasted Asparagus and Lemon Garlic Roasted Potatoes

Day 2:

- **Breakfast:** Avocado and Tomato Breakfast Sandwich
- **Lunch:** Lentil and Vegetable Soup with a side of Quinoa Tabbouleh
- **Dinner:** Quinoa-Stuffed Bell Peppers with Turkey and a side of Sesame Ginger Broccoli

Day 3:

- **Breakfast:** Blueberry Chia Pudding

- **Lunch:** Spinach and White Bean Soup with a side of Roasted Brussels Sprouts with Cranberries

- **Dinner:** Baked Salmon with Dill Sauce, served with Garlic Parmesan Mashed Cauliflower

Day 4:

- **Breakfast:** Banana Walnut Pancakes

- **Lunch:** Turkey and Quinoa Stew with a side of Balsamic Roasted Carrots

- **Dinner:** Spaghetti Squash with Pesto and Grilled Corn on the Cob with Chili-Lime Butter

Day 5:

- **Breakfast:** Zucchini and Feta Breakfast Muffins

- **Lunch:** Quinoa-Stuffed Mushrooms with a side of Spicy Cucumber Salad

- **Dinner:** Spinach and Feta Stuffed Chicken Breast with Sauteed Kale with Garlic

Day 6:

- **Breakfast:** Oatmeal with Almond Butter and Apples

- **Lunch:** Black Bean and Vegetable Stew with a side of Cilantro Lime Brown Rice

- **Dinner:** Ratatouille with Chickpeas served with Balsamic Roasted Brussels Sprouts

Day 7:

- **Breakfast:** Whole Wheat Banana Nut Waffles

- **Lunch:** Caprese Skewers with Balsamic Glaze and a side of Roasted Broccoli and Garlic

- **Dinner:** Shrimp and Quinoa Pilaf with Green Beans Almondine

<u>Week 2:</u>
Day 8:

- **Breakfast:** Cherry Almond Breakfast Bars

- **Lunch:** Greek Salad Bites with a side of Spicy Oven-Baked Sweet Potato Wedges

- **Dinner:** Baked Cod with Mediterranean Salsa and a side of Quinoa Tabbouleh

Day 9:

- **Breakfast:** Mango and Coconut Chia Pudding

- **Lunch:** Mexican Chicken and Vegetable Soup with a side of Roasted Garlic and White Bean Dip

- **Dinner:** Pesto Zucchini Noodles with Cherry Tomatoes and Grilled Lemon Dill Swordfish

Day 10:

- **Breakfast:** Whole Wheat Blueberry Muffins

- **Lunch:** Sweet Potato and Lentil Soup with a side of Lemon Herb Quinoa Pilaf

- **Dinner:** Quinoa and Black Bean Stuffed Bell Peppers with Turkey and a side of Roasted Brussels Sprouts with Cranberries

Day 11:

- **Breakfast:** Spinach and Mushroom Breakfast Quesadilla

- **Lunch:** Thai Red Curry Soup with a side of Garlic Parmesan Mashed Cauliflower

- **Dinner:** Chickpea and Vegetable Curry with Sautéed Spinach with Pine Nuts

Day 12:

- **Breakfast:** Banana and Walnut Breakfast Quinoa

- **Lunch:** Caprese Skewers with Balsamic Glaze and a side of Quinoa Tabbouleh

- **Dinner:** Lentil and Mushroom Meatballs with Cilantro Lime Brown Rice

Day 13:

- **Breakfast:** Greek Yogurt with Berries and Chia Seeds

- **Lunch:** Cucumber and Tomato Salsa with Baked Zucchini Fritters

- **Dinner:** Turkey and Sweet Potato Shepherd's Pie with a side of Sesame Ginger Broccoli

Day 14:

- **Breakfast:** Sweet Potato and Kale Breakfast Hash

- **Lunch:** Roasted Red Pepper Hummus with Spiced Edamame

- **Dinner:** Spaghetti Squash with Roasted Cherry Tomatoes and Grilled Corn on the Cob with Chili-Lime Butter

Week 3:

Day 15:

- **Breakfast:** Coconut Mango Smoothie Bowl

- **Lunch:** Roasted Garlic and White Bean Dip with Spicy Avocado Salsa

- **Dinner:** Grilled Lemon Herb Chicken with Roasted Asparagus and Lemon Garlic Roasted Potatoes

Day 16:

- **Breakfast:** Cinnamon Raisin Oatmeal with Sliced Apples

- **Lunch:** Creamy Broccoli and Potato Soup with a side of Balsamic Roasted Carrots

- **Dinner:** Spinach and Feta Stuffed Chicken Breast with Sautéed Kale with Garlic

Day 17:

- **Breakfast:** Smoked Salmon and Asparagus Frittata

- **Lunch:** Chickpea and Spinach Dip with Sliced Cucumbers

- **Dinner:** Quinoa-Stuffed Bell Peppers with Turkey and a side of Sesame Ginger Broccoli

Day 18:

- **Breakfast:** Banana Walnut Pancakes
- **Lunch:** Lentil and Vegetable Soup with a side of Quinoa Tabbouleh
- **Dinner:** Baked Salmon with Dill Sauce, served with Garlic Parmesan Mashed Cauliflower

Day 19:

- **Breakfast:** Mango and Coconut Chia Pudding
- **Lunch:** Caprese Skewers with Balsamic Glaze and a side of Roasted Broccoli and Garlic
- **Dinner:** Pesto Zucchini Noodles with Cherry Tomatoes and Grilled Lemon Dill Swordfish

Day 20:

- **Breakfast:** Greek Yogurt Parfait with Honey and Berries
- **Lunch:** Roasted Red Pepper Hummus with Zesty Cucumber Radish Salad
- **Dinner:** Ratatouille with Chickpeas served with Balsamic Roasted Brussels Sprouts

Day 21:

- **Breakfast:** Whole Wheat Blueberry Muffins
- **Lunch:** Cucumber and Tomato Salsa with Baked Zucchini Fritters
- **Dinner:** Shrimp and Quinoa Pilaf with Green Beans Almondine

Week 4:

Day 22:

- **Breakfast:** Banana and Walnut Breakfast Quinoa
- **Lunch:** Tuna Salad Lettuce Wraps with a side of Roasted Brussels Sprouts with Cranberries
- **Dinner:** Baked Cod with Mediterranean Salsa and a side of Quinoa Tabbouleh

Day 23:

- **Breakfast:** Blueberry Chia Pudding

- **Lunch:** Mexican Chicken and Vegetable Soup with a side of Spicy Oven-Baked Sweet Potato Wedges
- **Dinner:** Quinoa and Black Bean Stuffed Bell Peppers with Turkey and a side of Sautéed Spinach with Pine Nuts

Day 24:

- **Breakfast:** Spinach and Mushroom Frittata
- **Lunch:** Caprese Skewers with Balsamic Glaze and a side of Quinoa Tabbouleh
- **Dinner:** Lentil and Mushroom Meatballs with Cilantro Lime Brown Rice

Day 25:

- **Breakfast:** Zucchini and Feta Breakfast Muffins
- **Lunch:** Thai Red Curry Soup with a side of Garlic Parmesan Mashed Cauliflower
- **Dinner:** Ratatouille with Chickpeas served with Balsamic Roasted Brussels Sprouts

Day 26:

- **Breakfast:** Oatmeal with Almond Butter and Apples
- **Lunch:** Chickpea and Spinach Dip with Sliced Cucumbers
- **Dinner:** Grilled Lemon Herb Chicken with Roasted Asparagus and Lemon Garlic Roasted Potatoes

Day 27:

- **Breakfast:** Sweet Potato and Kale Breakfast Hash
- **Lunch:** Roasted Red Pepper Hummus with Spiced Edamame
- **Dinner:** Shrimp and Quinoa Pilaf with Green Beans Almondine

Day 28:

- **Breakfast:** Coconut Mango Smoothie Bowl
- **Lunch:** Cucumber and Tomato Salsa with Baked Zucchini Fritters
- **Dinner:** Pesto Zucchini Noodles with Cherry Tomatoes and Grilled Lemon Dill Swordfish

Week 5:

Day 29:

- **Breakfast:** Cherry Almond Breakfast Bars
- **Lunch:** Greek Salad Bites with a side of Roasted Broccoli and Garlic
- **Dinner:** Baked Salmon with Dill Sauce, served with Garlic Parmesan Mashed Cauliflower

Day 30:

- **Breakfast:** Mango and Coconut Chia Pudding
- **Lunch:** Lentil and Vegetable Soup with a side of Balsamic Roasted Carrots
- **Dinner:** Quinoa-Stuffed Bell Peppers with Turkey and a side of Sesame Ginger Broccoli

Day 31:

- **Breakfast:** Whole Wheat Blueberry Muffins
- **Lunch:** Caprese Skewers with Balsamic Glaze and a side of Quinoa Tabbouleh
- **Dinner:** Ratatouille with Chickpeas served with Balsamic Roasted Brussels Sprouts

Day 32:

- **Breakfast:** Spinach and Mushroom Breakfast Quesadilla
- **Lunch:** Thai Red Curry Soup with a side of Sautéed Spinach with Pine Nuts
- **Dinner:** Grilled Lemon Herb Chicken with Roasted Asparagus and Lemon Garlic Roasted Potatoes

Day 33:

- **Breakfast:** Banana Walnut Pancakes
- **Lunch:** Cucumber and Tomato Salsa with Zesty Cucumber Radish Salad
- **Dinner:** Shrimp and Quinoa Pilaf with Green Beans Almondine

Day 34:

- **Breakfast:** Greek Yogurt with Berries and Chia Seeds
- **Lunch:** Roasted Red Pepper Hummus with Spiced Edamame
- **Dinner:** Quinoa and Black Bean Stuffed Bell Peppers with Turkey and a side of Roasted Brussels Sprouts with Cranberries

Day 35:

- **Breakfast:** Sweet Potato and Kale Breakfast Hash
- **Lunch:** Tuna Salad Lettuce Wraps with a side of Quinoa Tabbouleh
- **Dinner:** Baked Cod with Mediterranean Salsa and a side of Garlic Parmesan Mashed Cauliflower

Week 6:

Day 36:

- **Breakfast:** Coconut Mango Smoothie Bowl
- **Lunch:** Chickpea and Spinach Dip with Sliced Cucumbers
- **Dinner:** Grilled Lemon Herb Chicken with Roasted Asparagus and Lemon Garlic Roasted Potatoes

Day 37:

- **Breakfast:** Banana and Walnut Breakfast Quinoa
- **Lunch:** Mexican Chicken and Vegetable Soup with a side of Roasted Garlic and White Bean Dip
- **Dinner:** Quinoa and Black Bean Stuffed Bell Peppers with Turkey and a side of Sautéed Spinach with Pine Nuts

Day 38:

- **Breakfast:** Spinach and Mushroom Frittata
- **Lunch:** Cucumber and Tomato Salsa with Baked Zucchini Fritters
- **Dinner:** Ratatouille with Chickpeas served with Balsamic Roasted Brussels Sprouts

Day 39:

- **Breakfast:** Blueberry Chia Pudding
- **Lunch:** Roasted Red Pepper Hummus with Zesty Cucumber Radish Salad
- **Dinner:** Lentil and Mushroom Meatballs with Cilantro Lime Brown Rice

Day 40:

- **Breakfast:** Zucchini and Feta Breakfast Muffins
- **Lunch:** Thai Red Curry Soup with a side of Garlic Parmesan Mashed Cauliflower
- **Dinner:** Baked Salmon with Dill Sauce, served with Garlic Parmesan Mashed Cauliflower

Day 41:

- **Breakfast:** Sweet Potato and Kale Breakfast Hash
- **Lunch:** Caprese Skewers with Balsamic Glaze and a side of Quinoa Tabbouleh
- **Dinner:** Shrimp and Quinoa Pilaf with Green Beans Almondine

Day 42:

- **Breakfast:** Greek Yogurt Parfait with Honey and Berries
- **Lunch:** Tuna Salad Lettuce Wraps with a side of Roasted Broccoli and Garlic
- **Dinner:** Quinoa-Stuffed Bell Peppers with Turkey and a side of Sesame Ginger Broccoli

Week 7:

Day 43:

- **Breakfast:** Cherry Almond Breakfast Bars
- **Lunch:** Greek Salad Bites with a side of Balsamic Roasted Carrots
- **Dinner:** Quinoa-Stuffed Bell Peppers with Turkey and a side of Sautéed Spinach with Pine Nuts

Day 44:

- **Breakfast:** Mango and Coconut Chia Pudding
- **Lunch:** Lentil and Vegetable Soup with a side of Quinoa Tabbouleh
- **Dinner:** Pesto Zucchini Noodles with Cherry Tomatoes and Grilled Lemon Dill Swordfish

Day 45:

- **Breakfast:** Whole Wheat Blueberry Muffins
- **Lunch:** Caprese Skewers with Balsamic Glaze and a side of Roasted Broccoli and Garlic
- **Dinner:** Ratatouille with Chickpeas served with Balsamic Roasted Brussels Sprouts

Day 46:

- **Breakfast:** Spinach and Mushroom Breakfast Quesadilla
- **Lunch:** Thai Red Curry Soup with a side of Garlic Parmesan Mashed Cauliflower
- **Dinner:** Grilled Lemon Herb Chicken with Roasted Asparagus and Lemon Garlic Roasted Potatoes

Day 47:

- **Breakfast:** Banana Walnut Pancakes
- **Lunch:** Cucumber and Tomato Salsa with Zesty Cucumber Radish Salad
- **Dinner:** Shrimp and Quinoa Pilaf with Green Beans Almondine

Day 48:

- **Breakfast:** Greek Yogurt with Berries and Chia Seeds
- **Lunch:** Roasted Red Pepper Hummus with Spiced Edamame
- **Dinner:** Baked Cod with Mediterranean Salsa and a side of Quinoa Tabbouleh

Day 49:

- **Breakfast:** Sweet Potato and Kale Breakfast Hash
- **Lunch:** Tuna Salad Lettuce Wraps with a side of Sesame Ginger Broccoli

- **Dinner:** Chicken and Vegetable Quinoa Soup with a side of Baked Zucchini Fritters

Week 8:

Day 50:

- **Breakfast:** Coconut Mango Smoothie Bowl

- **Lunch:** Chickpea and Spinach Dip with Sliced Cucumbers

- **Dinner:** Quinoa and Black Bean Stuffed Bell Peppers with Turkey and a side of Sautéed Spinach with Pine Nuts

Day 51:

- **Breakfast:** Banana and Walnut Breakfast Quinoa

- **Lunch:** Mexican Chicken and Vegetable Soup with a side of Roasted Garlic and White Bean Dip

- **Dinner:** Baked Salmon with Dill Sauce, served with Garlic Parmesan Mashed Cauliflower

Day 52:

- **Breakfast:** Spinach and Mushroom Frittata

- **Lunch:** Cucumber and Tomato Salsa with Baked Zucchini Fritters

- **Dinner:** Ratatouille with Chickpeas served with Balsamic Roasted Brussels Sprouts

Day 53:

- **Breakfast:** Blueberry Chia Pudding

- **Lunch:** Roasted Red Pepper Hummus with Zesty Cucumber Radish Salad

- **Dinner:** Lentil and Mushroom Meatballs with Cilantro Lime Brown Rice

Day 54:

- **Breakfast:** Zucchini and Feta Breakfast Muffins

- **Lunch:** Thai Red Curry Soup with a side of Garlic Parmesan Mashed Cauliflower

- **Dinner:** Grilled Lemon Herb Chicken with Roasted Asparagus and Lemon Garlic Roasted Potatoes

Day 55:

- **Breakfast:** Sweet Potato and Kale Breakfast Hash

- **Lunch:** Caprese Skewers with Balsamic Glaze and a side of Quinoa Tabbouleh

- **Dinner:** Shrimp and Quinoa Pilaf with Green Beans Almondine

Day 56:

- **Breakfast:** Greek Yogurt Parfait with Honey and Berries

- **Lunch:** Tuna Salad Lettuce Wraps with a side of Roasted Broccoli and Garlic

- **Dinner:** Quinoa-Stuffed Bell Peppers with Turkey and a side of Sesame Ginger Broccoli

Chapter 10: DASH Diet Grocery Shopping List

Creating a DASH Diet-friendly kitchen starts with a carefully planned grocery shopping list. This guide aims to help you select a variety of nutritious ingredients, which can be used to prepare heart-healthy and delicious meals. Create a shopping list that includes the essential components of the DASH Diet, which emphasizes a well-rounded mix of nutrients and flavors.

1. Fresh Produce:

- Leafy Greens (Spinach, Kale, Swiss Chard)
- Colorful Bell Peppers
- Tomatoes (Fresh and Canned)
- Cucumbers
- Avocados
- Berries (Blueberries, Strawberries, Raspberries)
- Apples
- Oranges and Grapefruits
- Bananas

2. Whole Grains:

- Brown Rice
- Quinoa
- Whole Wheat Pasta
- Oats (Old-Fashioned or Steel-Cut)
- Barley
- Farro

- Whole Grain Bread

3. Lean Proteins:

- Skinless Chicken Breast
- Lean Ground Turkey or Chicken
- Salmon or Trout
- Lentils
- Chickpeas
- Tofu
- Eggs

4. Dairy or Dairy Alternatives:

- Low-Fat Greek Yogurt
- Skim or Low-Fat Milk
- Feta or Goat Cheese (in moderation)
- Almond or Soy Milk (unsweetened)

5. Healthy Fats:

- Extra Virgin Olive Oil
- Avocado Oil

- Nuts (Almonds, Walnuts, Pistachios)
- Seeds (Chia, Flaxseed, Pumpkin Seeds)
- Avocados

6. Fresh Herbs and Spices:

- Basil
- Oregano
- Thyme
- Cumin
- Turmeric
- Garlic
- Ginger
- Rosemary
- Dill

7. Whole Vegetables and Starchy Vegetables:

- Sweet Potatoes
- Carrots
- Zucchini
- Butternut Squash
- Beets
- Corn (fresh or frozen)

8. Canned and Dried Goods:

- Low-Sodium Canned Beans (Kidney, Black, Cannellini)
- Diced Tomatoes (No Added Salt)
- Tomato Paste
- Low-Sodium Chicken or Vegetable Broth
- Whole Grain Cereal (Low in Sugar)
- Quinoa or Brown Rice Flour

9. Beverages:

- Green Tea
- Herbal Teas (No Added Sugar)
- Sparkling Water (No Added Sugar)
- Freshly Squeezed Citrus Juices

10. Snacks:

- Hummus
- Whole Grain Crackers
- Raw Vegetables for Snacking
- Air-Popped Popcorn (Plain)

11. Condiments and Sauces:

- Balsamic Vinegar
- Dijon Mustard
- Salsa (Low Sodium)
- Herbs and Spices for Seasoning

12. Frozen Foods:

- Frozen Berries

- Mixed Vegetables (No Added Sauce)
- Skinless, Boneless Fish Fillets

With this DASH Diet Grocery Shopping List, you'll have a helpful guide to confidently navigate the aisles and select heart-healthy ingredients for your culinary journey. Embrace the variety of colors and nutrient-rich choices, and get ready to create delicious meals that nourish your body and delight your taste buds. Have a pleasant shopping experience!

Chapter 11

Portion Control & Efficient Meal Prep Tips

Portion control and balanced Nutrition

The DASH Diet not only recommends what to eat but also emphasizes portion sizes. Portion control is an important aspect of the DASH approach, which emphasizes balanced nutrition and helps prevent excessive calorie intake. By maintaining a balanced intake of carbohydrates, proteins, and fats, you can ensure that your body receives the necessary nutrients without consuming excessive amounts, which can help with weight management and overall health.

When exploring the DASH Diet Basics, it's important to understand that it is more than just a short-term dietary change. It is a long-term lifestyle that supports heart health and overall well-being. By understanding the principles that guide the DASH Diet, you can make informed and nutritious choices that align with your body's needs. Prepare yourself for a journey towards improved health and well-being!

Efficient Meal Prep Tips

Efficiency in the kitchen can be helpful when following the DASH Diet. These meal prep tips can help simplify your cooking routine and make it easier to include heart-healthy choices in your daily meals.

1. **Batch Cook Staples:** Prepare larger quantities of foundational elements like quinoa, brown rice, and grilled chicken for batch cooking. Store the ingredients in portioned containers so that they are ready to be used in different meals during the week. This not only saves time but helps ensure that you always have nutritious essentials readily available.

2. **Pre-Chop Vegetables:** Take some time to prepare your vegetables ahead of time. Wash, chop, and store the ingredients in containers so they are prepared for easy use in salads, stir-fries, and snacks. Having a variety of colorful vegetables readily available can help you incorporate them more often into your DASH Diet meals.

3. **Prepare Snacks in Advance:** Separate snacks such as nuts, fruits, and yogurt into individual portions. This not only helps with portion control

but also makes it easy to grab a healthy snack when feeling hungry. Having pre-portioned snacks can help you stay on track with your DASH Diet goals.

4. **Select Versatile Ingredients:** Choose ingredients that can be used in multiple ways for various meals. For example, roasted vegetables can be served as a side dish during dinner and then added to a salad for lunch. Strategic planning aims to optimize ingredient usage and reduce waste.

5. **Prepare Mason Jar Salads:** Assemble salads in mason jars, stack ingredients in the right order, starting with the wet ones and ending with the dry ones. This method helps to keep the salad from getting soggy, and it's convenient to have a jar ready for a fast and healthy meal. Try different combinations of vegetables and proteins to keep your salads interesting.

6. **Use Slow Cookers and Instant Pots:** Make use of time-saving cooking appliances such as slow cookers and Instant Pots. These devices can help you prepare delicious and nutritious meals with little effort. Prepare the dish, leave it to cook, and come back to find a perfectly cooked meal that adheres to the DASH Diet.

7. **Keep a Variety of DASH Diet-Friendly Sauces:** Have a selection of DASH Diet-approved sauces on hand to enhance flavors without needing to use too much salt. You can make your own salsa, hummus, and yogurt-based dressings to add flavor to your meals. These options are also good for your heart health.

8. **Create Freezer-Friendly Dishes:** To make things easier, you can cook larger amounts of DASH Diet recipes and then freeze them in individual portions. This helps to ensure that you always have a nutritious meal available, even on your busiest days. Soups, stews, and casseroles are excellent options for freezing.

9. **Pre-Portion Smoothie Ingredients:** To prepare convenient and healthy breakfasts or snacks, pre-portion smoothie ingredients in freezer bags. Include fruits, vegetables, and any other desired add-ins. In the morning, blend with your preferred liquid for a refreshing smoothie that is packed with nutrients.

10. **Take Out a Day for Meal Prep:** Designate a specific day each week for meal prep. Make use of this time to plan your meals, chop ingredients, and organize your refrigerator. Following this proactive approach will help you maintain adherence to the DASH Diet throughout the week.

By incorporating these quick and easy meal prep tips into your routine, you'll discover that following the DASH Diet is not only good for your health but also saves you time and is enjoyable. Simplifying how you prepare your meals can help you have a week full of tasty, healthy, and good-for-your-heart dishes

Chapter 12: Frequently Asked Questions and Troubleshooting

Starting a DASH Diet journey can lead to questions and occasional challenges. This chapter is designed to help you with common questions and provide solutions to potential challenges, so you can easily incorporate the DASH Diet into your daily life.

Frequently Asked Questions about the DASH Diet

Can I eat out while following the DASH Diet? Yes! When dining out, consider choosing restaurants that offer a variety of menu options, including lean proteins, whole grains, and plenty of vegetables. Remember to pay attention to portion sizes and consider requesting modifications to align with DASH principles.

Is alcohol allowed on the DASH Diet? Moderation is key. While the DASH Diet does not have specific restrictions on alcohol, it is recommended to consume it in moderation. Choose heart-healthy options such as red wine and be cautious of the amount of added sugars in cocktails.

How can I manage my sodium intake? Reducing sodium is a vital component of the DASH Diet. Choose fresh, whole foods instead of processed options, enhance taste with herbs and spices, and be mindful of hidden sources of sodium. Gradually reduce the amount of salt in recipes to help your taste buds adjust.

Can I modify the DASH Diet to fit my dietary preferences? Sure. The DASH Diet can be adapted to different dietary preferences, such as vegetarian, vegan, or gluten-free. Make sure to include nutrient-rich options in your diet to meet your nutritional requirements.

Overcoming Challenges and Staying Committed

1. **Managing Time Constraints:** Create a plan based on priorities. Use time-saving techniques such as batch cooking, meal prepping, and relying on quick recipes. The DASH Diet can be adapted to different schedules with proper planning.

2. **Addressing Flavor Boredom:** To combat flavor boredom, try experimenting with herbs, spices, and new recipes. The DASH Diet

promotes culinary creativity, giving you the opportunity to experiment with various flavors while following its guidelines. Rotate your food choices to keep your taste buds stimulated.

3. **Managing Social Situations:** Politely communicate your dietary preferences. Many social gatherings provide a range of food options, giving you the opportunity to make conscious decisions. If possible, bring a nutritious DASH-friendly dish along to share with everyone.

4. **Dealing with Weight Loss Plateaus:** Consider reassessing your portion sizes and overall calorie intake. Include additional physical activity in your daily routine and think about seeking guidance from a healthcare professional or nutritionist for personalized recommendations.

By navigating the frequently asked questions and troubleshooting potential challenges, you can gain confidence in embracing the DASH Diet. This chapter provides guidance to help you have a successful and enjoyable journey towards heart-healthy living. Embrace the flexibility of the DASH Diet and make it a sustainable and enriching part of your lifestyle.

Conclusion

This DASH Diet journey has helped you move towards improved health while enjoying delicious and nutritious meals along the way. The principles of the Dietary Approaches to Stop Hypertension (DASH) diet have guided your food choices and have also influenced your holistic approach to well-being.

The DASH Diet is more than just a set of guidelines. It's an invitation to adopt a heart-healthy lifestyle. By understanding the basic principles of the DASH Diet, incorporating necessary kitchen tools and ingredients, and becoming proficient in meal planning and preparation, you have established a strong basis for long-term well-being.

This cookbook presents a variety of recipes that highlight the diversity and flavor of the DASH Diet. Each recipe in this book showcases the abundance of whole, nutrient-dense foods, ranging from energizing breakfasts to satisfying dinners and delightful snacks.

The FAQs and troubleshooting chapter provides you with the necessary knowledge to navigate common queries and challenges effectively. With the tools provided, you can now stay committed to your heart-healthy journey by managing sodium intake, customizing the DASH Diet according to dietary preferences, and overcoming time constraints.

The DASH Diet is a sustainable lifestyle, rather than a temporary fix. The meal prep tips provided aim to make healthy eating both achievable and convenient. Batch cooking, prepping ingredients, and using time-saving appliances can help make the DASH Diet more accessible and enjoyable as part of your routine.

As you conclude this cookbook, remember that your journey with the DASH Diet continues. Keep exploring new recipes, experimenting with flavors, and staying attentive to the needs of your body. Utilize the knowledge acquired here to make informed decisions that enhance your overall well-being.

In conclusion, this cookbook celebrates not only the end of a culinary journey but also the start of a heart-healthy lifestyle. Here's to a future filled with good health, delicious meals, and the happiness that comes from nourishing your body with the nutrients it deserves. May the principles of the DASH Diet continue to guide and inspire you on your journey towards a heart-healthy and fulfilling life.

Recipe Index

W

Watermelon and Feta Skewers 55

Whole Wheat Banana Nut Waffles 25

Whole Wheat Blueberry Muffins 39

Z

Zesty Cucumber Radish Salad 57

Zucchini and Feta Breakfast Muffins 16